Editor
Anne Grete Semb

Handbook of Cardiovascular Disease Management in Rheumatoid Arthritis

Editor

Anne Grete Semb, MD, PhD
Preventive Cardio-Rheuma Clinic
Dept of Rheumatology
Diakonhjemmet hospital
Oslo, Norway

Handbook of Cardiovascular Disease Management in Rheumatoid Arthritis

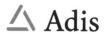

Editor

Anne Grete Semb MD, PhD
Preventive Cardio-Rheuma Clinic
Dept of Rheumatology
Diakonhjemmet hospital
Oslo
Norway

Contributors

Carolyn A Ball, MD
Cynthia S Crowson, MS
Theodoros Dimitroulas, MD, PhD
Sherine E Gabriel, MD, MSc
Eirik Ikdahl, MD
George Kitas, MD, PhD, FRCP
Rekha Mankad, MD, FACC
Eric L Matteson, MD, MPH
Elena Myasoedova, MD, PhD
Stephen Nicholls, MD, PhD
Silvia Rollefstad, MD, PhD
Anne Grete Semb, MD, PhD
Piet van Riel, MD, PhD

ISBN 978-3-319-26780-7   ISBN 978-3-319-26782-1 (eBook)
DOI 10.1007/978-3-319-26782-1

Printed on acid-free paper

This Adis imprint is published by Springer Nature
The registered company is Springer International Publishing AG Switzerland

Project editor: Laura Hajba

Contents

Editor and author biographies

Anne Grete Semb, MD, PhD is a senior consultant cardiologist, the founder and leader of a Preventive Cardio-Rheuma Clinic, the leader of the cardiovascular-rheuma research team at Dept of Rheumatology, Diakonhjemmet hospital, Oslo, Norway and has 8 PhD students. She is a regular reviewer for several international rheumatology and cardiology journals. She has published more than 200 original scientific publications in peer-reviewed journals, book chapters and conference abstracts. She has led 3 clinical trials/studies, participated in 17 clinical trials/studies, whereas 13 trials/studies have been investigator initiated. She is a member of the European Society of Cardiology (ESC) Working Group of Cardiovascular Pharmacology and Drug Therapy. She is a member of the Eular task force group for Cardiovascular Disease Risk Management in Rheumatic Diseases in 2010 and 2015, one of the founders of and now the administrative leader of the A TransAtlantic Cardiovascular risk Consortium for Rheumatoid Arthritis (ATACC-RA).

Caroline Ball, MD is a fellow in cardiovascular diseases at Loyola University Medical Center in Maywood, IL, USA. She completed her residency in internal medicine at Mayo Clinic, Rochester, MN, USA. She received her MD with distinction in research from Loyola University Chicago Stritch School of Medicine. Her clinical interests include preventive cardiology, heart disease in women, and heart disease in patients with rheumatologic conditions.

Cynthia S Crowson, MS is Associate Professor of Medicine and Assistant Professor of Biostatistics at Mayo Clinic, Rochester, Minnesota, USA. She has a Master's degree in Statistics from Iowa State University. Her research interests are focused on performing statistical analyses to further the study of rheumatologic diseases, with an emphasis on epidemiologic studies and cardiovascular disease outcomes. Her statistical research interests have recently been focused on assessment of calibration of prognostic risk scores. She currently serves on the editorial boards of several rheumatology journals.

Theodoros Dimitroulas, MD, PhD earned his medical degree (1999), master's degree in medical methodology (2005) and PhD in medicine (2009) from Aristotle University of Thessaloniki, Greece and is currently an Assistant Professor in Rheumatology at this institution. He worked as Consultant Rheumatologist in the UK (2010-2015) and during this period he investigated the role of specific biomarkers in the development of endothelial dysfunction in rheumatoid arthritis. Apart from this field his other scientific interests include pulmonary hypertension in connective tissue diseases and the clinical applications of musculoskeletal ultrasound.

Sherine E Gabriel, MD, MSc is Professor & Dean, Rutgers Robert Wood Johnson Medical School and CEO of the Robert Wood Johnson Medical Group. She is also Dean Emerita, Mayo Medical School and the former, William J and Charles H Mayo Endowed Professor. Dr Gabriel is past president of the American College of Rheumatology. Dr Gabriel earned a Doctor of Medicine degree, with distinction, from the University of Saskatchewan, Canada and completed Internal Medicine Residency and Rheumatology fellowship at Mayo Graduate School of Medicine. She then earned a Master of Science in Clinical Epidemiology from McMaster University. She is certified by the American Board of Internal Medicine in Internal Medicine and in Rheumatology. Dr Gabriel's research, which is largely NIH funded, has resulted in >250 peer-reviewed, original scientific publications addressing the epidemiology of the rheumatic diseases with an emphasis on cardiovascular comorbidity.

Eirik Ikdahl, MD, is a PhD student at the Preventive Cardio-Rheuma Clinic, Department of Rheumatology, Diakonhjemmet Hospital, Oslo, Norway. Ikdahl holds a medical degree from the University of Oslo, 2014, and has been involved in rheumatology research at Diakonhjemmet Hospital since 2009. His main areas of research include vascular biomarkers and cardio-rheuma epidemiology projects. Ikdahl is currently the daily leader of the NOrwegian Collaboration on the Atherosclerosis in patients with Rheumatic joint diseases (The NOCAR) project, which is a Norwegian nationwide project including 11 rheumatology outpatient hospital centres. He has published 7 papers, 38 abstracts and 4 chapters in books/reviews.

George Kitas, MD, PhD, FRCP is Consultant Rheumatologist and Head of Research and Development at the Dudley Group NHS Foundation Trust in the UK. He leads the Rheumatoid Arthritis Comorbidity Research Group, has authored >320 PubMed-listed papers (about 200 in the field of cardiovascular comorbidity of RA). He is Convenor of the British Society for Rheumatology Cardiovascular Comorbidity Special Interest Group and member of the EULAR task force for recommendations on Cardiovascular Risk Management in Inflammatory Joint Disease.

Rekha Mankad, MD, FACC is Assistant Professor of Medicine, Mayo Clinic College of Medicine, Rochester Minnesota, USA, and is a consultant in the Division of Cardiovascular Diseases. Dr Mankad is the Director of the Cardio-Rheumatology Clinic and works within the Women's Heart Clinic and Valvular Heart Disease Clinic. Dr. Mankad received her MD degree from the Northeast Ohio Medical University. Her clinical interest has been in the field of women and heart disease as well as the new arena of cardiovascular disease in the rheumatologic patient. As Director of the Cardio-Rheumatology Clinic, Dr Mankad, in conjunction with her rheumatology colleagues, is working on addressing the risk factors and treatment options for the patient with rheumatologic conditions who are known to be at increased cardiovascular risk.

Eric L Matteson, MD, MPH, is Professor of Medicine, Mayo Clinic College of Medicine, Rochester, Minnesota, USA, and Chair Emeritus, Division of Rheumatology with joint appointment in the Division of Epidemiology in the Department of Health Sciences Research. Dr Matteson received his MD degree from Friedrich-Alexander University at Erlangen-Nuremberg. Dr Matteson's clinical and research interests are in the fields of inflammatory arthritis and vasculitis. His research agenda includes investigation into the epidemiology of these diseases and their clinical disease expression and effect on patients who suffer from them, systemic manifestations of rheumatologic disease, biomarkers of disease susceptibility and disease activity, and clinical trials of novel agents.

Elena Myasoedova, MD, PhD is a Rheumatologist, Assistant Professor of Internal Medicine at Mayo Clinic College of Medicine (Rochester, MN, USA). Dr Myasoedova has completed her medical education in Russia, where she earned her MD degree with distinction, a PhD degree, a Doctor of Medical Sciences degree and completed her training in Internal Medicine and Rheumatology. In 2008 she came to Mayo Clinic as a Fulbright scholar and has been working on clinical epidemiology research in the field of rheumatoid arthritis pertaining to cardiovascular diseases and other comorbidities, focusing on the approaches to improve outcomes of patients with rheumatoid arthritis. She completed her residency in Internal Medicine at Mayo Clinic, Rochester, MN, USA and is currently a Clinical Fellow at the Division of Rheumatology at Mayo Clinic, Rochester, MN.

Silvia Rollefstad, MD, PhD is currently working as a physician and post doc researcher at the Preventive Cardio-Rheuma clinic, Department of Rheumatology, Diakonhjemmet Hospital, Oslo, Norway. Her major research activities have been in the interdisciplinary field of cardiology and rheumatology. Dr Rollefstad has 16 Pubmed-indexed publications (H-index: 5), and is in the writing committee for the update of the EULAR recommendations for management of cardiovascular disease in patients with inflammatory joint diseases.

Abbreviations

AA	Amyloid A
AAA	Ask, Advice, and Act approach
ACC	American College of Cardiology
ACE	Angiotensin-converting enzyme
ACPA	Anti-citrullinated peptide antibody
ACS	Acute coronary syndrome
AF	Atrial fibrillation
AHA	American Heart Association
ApoB:ApoA	Apolipoprotein B:apolipoprotein A
ARB	Angiotensin receptor blocker
AV	Atrioventricular
BB	Beta-blocker
bDMARDs	Biologic disease-modifying antirheumatic drugs
BMI	Body mass index
BP	Blood pressure
BRM	Biologic response modifiers
CABG	Coronary artery bypass grafting
CAD	Coronary artery disease
CDAI	Clinical disease activity index;
CIRAS	Claims-based index of RA severity;
CHD	Coronary heart disease
CI	Confidence interval
c-IMT	Carotid intima-media thickness
CK	Creatine kinase
CKD	Chronic kidney disease
CMR	Cardiac magnetic resonance
COMORA	Comorbidities in RA
CP	Carotid plaques
CRP	C-reactive protein
CVD	Cardiovascular disease
DBP	Diastolic blood pressure
DM	Diabetes mellitus

EAS	European Atherosclerosis Society
ECGs	Electrocardiograms
EF	Ejection fraction
ER	Edema ratio
ERS-RA	Expanded Cardiovascular Risk Prediction Score for Rheumatoid Arthritis
ESC	European Society of Cardiology
ESR	Erythrocyte sedimentation rate
ESRD	End-stage renal disease
EULAR	European League Against Rheumatism
ExRA	Extra articular disease manifestations of RA
FRS	Framingham risk score
HbA1c	Blood glucose/glycated hemoglobin
HDL-c	High-density lipoprotein cholesterol
HFPEF	Heart failure with preserved ejection fraction
HRV	Heart rate variability
HZ	Hazard ratio
JUPITER	Justification for the Use of statins in primary Prevention: an Intervention Trial Evaluating Rosuvastatin
IL-1	Interleukin 1
IMR	Incidence mortality rates
IMT	Intima-media thickness
ISH	Isolated systolic hypertension
LGE	Late gadolinium enhancement
LDL-c	Low density lipoprotein cholesterol
LV	Left ventricular
LVH	Left ventricular hypertrophy
MI	Myocardial infarction
NBTE	Nonbacterial thrombotic endocarditis
NCEP	National Cholesterol Education Program
NO	Nitric oxide
NOAR	Norfolk Arthritis Register
NSAIDs	Non-steroidal anti-inflammatory drugs
OR	Odds ratio

OxLDL	Oxidized low-density lipoproteins
PCI	Percutaneous coronary intervention
PCSK9	Proprotein convertase subtilisin/kexin type 9 inhibitors
PWD	P-wave dispersion
QRISK2	QRESEARCH Cardiovascular Risk Algorithm 2
QTc	Corrected QT interval
RA	Rheumatoid arthritis
RARBIS	Records-based index of severity;
RF	Rheumatoid factor
ROS	Reactive oxygen species
RR	Relative risk
RV	Rheumatoid vasculitis
SBP	Systolic blood pressure
SCD	Sudden cardiac death
SCORE	Systematic COronary Risk Evaluation
SDAI	Simplified disease activity index
SMR	Standardized mortality rate
TC	Total cholesterol
Th	T-helper lymphocytes
TIA	Transient ischemic attack
TNF	Tumor necrosis factor
TNF-i	Tumour necrosis factor inhibitor
TRACE-RA	TRial of Atorvastatin for the primary prevention of Cardiovascular Events in patients with Rheumatoid Arthritis
TTE	Transthoracic echocardiography
VCAM	Vascular cell adhesion molecule
VHD	Valvular heart disease
WHO	World Health Organization

Preface

Over the course of the last 30 years, cardiovascular disease (CVD) morbidity and mortality rates in the Western world have progressively declined on the basis of more intensive prevention approaches aimed at smoking cessation and lowering levels of cholesterol and blood pressure. However, there remains a considerable residual risk of clinical events with CVD continuing to be the most common cause of death in most countries. Accordingly, there is an ongoing need to identify additional targets for therapeutic intervention in order to achieve more effective prevention of one of the world's major public health problems.

During the same period of time, seminal insights from pathology and clinical studies have characterized a pivotal role for inflammation in the pathogenesis of CVD. Cellular and humoral mediators of inflammation have been implicated in the formation, progression and clinical expression of a broad range of CVD disorders including the vasculature, myocardium, and pericardium. As a result, there has been increasing interest in the development of inflammation-related biomarkers for diagnosis and risk prediction, and targeted anti-inflammatory therapies for both disease prevention and treatment.

As the role of inflammation in CVD has been increasingly elucidated, there has been considerable interest focused on the CVD manifestations of a range of systemic inflammatory diseases. In particular, an abundant body of literature has now demonstrated clear associations between rheumatoid arthritis (RA) and CVD, both commonly encountered conditions worldwide. Recent studies have demonstrated that the presence of RA portends a high CVD risk, comparable to that observed in the setting of diabetes mellitus. Subsequent efforts have attempted to define the most effective approaches to reducing CVD risk in RA patients, whether that be via use of RA-targeted therapies or by intensification of conventional CVD prevention strategies. Small clinical studies have provided important insights, although larger trials are urgently needed.

Semb and colleagues have presented an elegant overview of the role of rheumatoid arthritis in a broad range of CVD disorders. They comprehensively review the evidence spanning from studies of biological samples and populations through to the clinical bedside. It provides the reader with a contemporary analysis of what is known and what remains to be further clarified. It represents an important compilation of the literature by a star-studded group of clinical investigators in the field. It will further stimulate us to identify better ways to prevent the alarmingly high CVD risk observed in RA. To many, inflammation remains the next frontier as a target for modification in CVD. RA represents the prototype from which our foray continues beyond this frontier. As a result, this book provides a great road map for that journey.

Stephen Nicholls, MD, PhD
Adelaide
July 2016

Chapter 1

Overview of rheumatoid arthritis and mortality in relation to cardiovascular disease

Elena Myasoedova and Sherine E Gabriel

Global burden of rheumatoid arthritis: trends in incidence, prevalence, and mortality

Rheumatoid arthritis (RA) is a chronic destructive autoimmune disease with significant, often debilitating joint involvement, associated extra-articular manifestations, excess comorbidity and increased mortality. Incidence and prevalence of RA in populations varies substantially between geographic areas and over time [1–8]. The vast majority of studies report RA epidemiology in western high-income countries including Western Europe and North America. RA disease burden in low- and middle-income countries, in particularly in the Eastern populations, is less known, thus limiting the understanding of worldwide RA epidemiology.

Incidence of rheumatoid arthritis

A systematic review by Alamanos et al summarizing literature data on RA epidemiology from 1988 through 2005 has reported the median annual RA incidence rates for several major areas of the world, including North America (median 38; range 31–45 cases/100000 population); Northern European countries (median 29; range 24–36 cases/100000); Southern European countries (median 16.5; range 9–24 cases/100000) [1]. In all

© Springer International Publishing Switzerland 2017
A.G. Semb (ed.), *Handbook of Cardiovascular Disease Management in Rheumatoid Arthritis*, DOI 10.1007/978-3-319-26782-1_1

geographic areas, females were more likely to develop RA than men. The incidence studies for RA in developing countries are lacking.

Despite the variability of RA incidence rates in different populations at various time points, trends in RA incidence in different countries during the past several decades seems to follow a similar pattern. Indeed, a number of studies from different countries reported declines in RA incidence during the second half of the 20th century [3–8]. In particular, in Olmsted County, Minnesota, the incidence of RA in the adult population fell progressively from 61.2/100,000 in 1955–1964 to 32.7/100000 in 1985–1994 (we refer to data from this cohort in greater detail throughout this chapter) [6].

The more recent RA incidence trends are much less known. A Medicare-based analysis of age-associated diseases, including RA, did not show significant change in RA incidence during the 1992–2005 period in elderly US females [9]. From Olmsted County, Minnesota, there has been reported a modest increase in RA incidence among women during the period from 1995 to 2007 (by 2.5%/year from 1995 to 2007; 95% confidence interval [CI] 0.3%, 4.7%/year, p=0.02), but not in men (0.5% decrease/year; 95% CI: −3.6%–2.7%; p=0.74) [10]. This increase was found to be similar among all age groups. The overall age- and sex-adjusted annual RA incidence among the residents of Olmsted County, Minnesota ≥18 years for the 1995–2007 period was 40.9/100000 (95% CI 37.2–44.7). The age-adjusted incidence in women was 53.1/100000 (95% CI 47.3–58.9), and in men was: 27.7/100000 (95% CI 23.1–32.2).

Prevalence of rheumatoid arthritis

Concordantly with RA incidence rates, the prevalence of RA has varied depending on geographical area and calendar time. The lowest median estimates have been reported in Southern European countries (0.33%) and developing countries (0.35%), followed by Northern European countries (0.5%) [1]. The highest prevalence has been reported in the US population from Olmsted County, Minnesota: 1%, as estimated on 1/1/1985 with a decline to 0.62% by 1995 [4,10], concordant with decline in RA prevalence as reported in other populations [5,8]. In the following years, the prevalence of RA in this population increased to 0.72% by 2005.

However, this increase was confined to increasing prevalence in women (0.98% in 2005), but not in men, reflecting the increase in incidence rates in this population as described above [10]. These estimates can be applied to the US 2005 population suggesting an overall prevalence of 1.5 million US adults affected by RA in 2005 [10].

The understanding of the global burden of RA has been significantly advanced by the recent initiative 'Global Burden of Disease 2010 study' (GBD 2010). The GBD 2010 was a comprehensive effort to measure epidemiological levels and trends of 291 diseases, including musculoskeletal conditions and particularly RA, in 187 countries [11]. By applying a systematic review approach to the existing data on RA epidemiology and using statistical modeling, including disease-relevant country characteristics and random effects for each country and territory with little or no data on RA epidemiology, the study was able to predict RA prevalence and mortality globally including countries and regions with missing RA epidemiology data.

Of the 291 conditions studied in the GBD 2010 Study, RA was ranked 74th in terms of burden as measured by disability-adjusted life years. The estimated global prevalence of RA diagnosed based on the 1987 ACR criteria, for all age groups (5–100 years of age) in 2010 was 0.24% (95% CI 0.23%–0.25%), with the major peak of RA prevalence occurring in older ages (Figure 1.1).

The global prevalence remained stable from 1990 to 2010. The prevalence in women was approximately twofold higher than in men (mean 0.35% versus 0.13%, respectively), with no significant change from 1990 to 2010 for either sex. Modeled age-standardized prevalence in 2010 was highest in the Australasian region (mean 0.46%), Western Europe, and North America (mean 0.44% for both); and lowest in East and Southeast Asia and North Africa/Middle East (mean 0.16% for all).

In summary, the epidemiological burden of RA remains significant with stable global prevalence estimates, suggesting a continued societal burden associated with this disease. Despite sharp decline in RA incidence over the past four decades, there may be an increase in RA prevalence in some populations suggesting a possibility of impeding increase in the overall RA burden in the upcoming years. More studies are warranted to understand the recent trends in RA incidence worldwide in order to better address health care planning and delivery.

Mortality in rheumatoid arthritis

Since it was first described by Cobb and colleagues in 1953, the evidence for the disproportionately increased mortality in patients with RA has

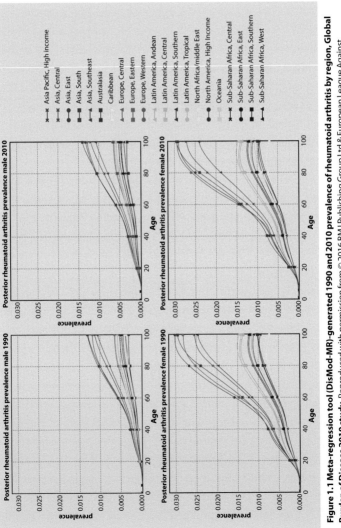

Figure 1.1 Meta-regression tool (DisMod-MR)-generated 1990 and 2010 prevalence of rheumatoid arthritis by region, Global Burden of Disease 2010 study. Reproduced with permission from © 2016 BMJ Publishing Group Ltd & European League Against Rheumatism, 2014. All Rights Reserved. Cross et al [11].

been accumulating worldwide. It is recognized that RA patients have had ~50% increased risk of premature mortality, and their life expectancy has been decreased by 3–10 years compared with the general population. These data underscore the need to target mortality in RA.

In contrast with the dramatic secular declines in overall mortality rates for the general population, the differences between observed and expected mortality in RA have increased substantially over time [12]. This resulted in a widening mortality gap between patients with RA, particularly rheumatoid factor (RF)-positive RA, and the general population (Figure 1.2) [13].

This phenomenon was first described in 2007 in the population-based incidence RA cohort from Olmsted County, Minnesota. Later, a similar trend toward a widening mortality gap between RA and non-RA subjects was shown in a European population, where no improvement in survival in RA was found in the past two decades [14].

Indeed, up until the mid-1990s there has been no consistent evidence for significant reduction in mortality in individual studies from different RA populations worldwide [12–16]. However, a declining trend in mortality in RA has been detected in a recent meta-analysis summarizing

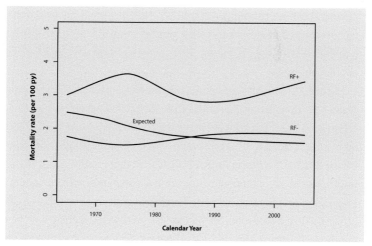

Figure 1.2 Observed and expected mortality in patients with rheumatoid factor-positive (RF+) and rheumatoid factor-negative (RF−) rheumatoid arthritis. Expected mortality is based on the Minnesota Caucasian population. Reproduced with permission from © The Journal of Rheumatology, 2008. All Rights Reserved. Gonzalez et al [13].

11 longitudinal studies on RA mortality over the past five decades [17]. Comparing pooled incidence mortality rates (IMR) the authors found a significant decrease in IMRs from 4.7/100 patient-years in studies done before 1970 to 2.0/100 patient-years in studies after 1983 (p<0.01). In addition, they found a relative decrease in RA mortality of 2.6%/year between 1955 and 1995. However, no decrease in the standardized mortality ratios (SMR) has been found (meta-SMR 2.01), suggesting that mortality in RA remains substantially elevated compared with the general population [17].

Since 1995, there has been growing evidence that mortality in RA patients is declining. A significant decrease in overall mortality in RA patients diagnosed since 1995 compared with those diagnosed in the earlier decades has been reported in Olmsted County, Minnesota [18]. The 5-year mortality estimate was 6.6% in the 1995–2007 incidence RA cohort compared with 12.9% in the 1985–1994 incidence cohort. Survival trends were similar in both genders and in both RF-positive and RF-negative patients. Likewise, a declining mortality trend from 1996 to 2009 has been reported in RA patients from a Canadian population with SMR ranging from 13.0 deaths/1000 RA patients in 1996 to 9.2 deaths/1000 RA patients in 2009 [19]. Notably, the authors reported an unchanged relative mortality gap between RA and the general population with approximately 50% increased mortality in RA versus non-RA subjects.

A Norfolk Arthritis Register (NOAR) study reported a decline in crude seven-year overall mortality rates from 21.3/1000 person years in a RA cohort who were first enrolled in the register in 1990–1994 to 20.0/1000 person years in a RA cohort who were first enrolled in 2000–2004 based on the 2010 ACR criteria for RA [20]. The authors found no significant improvement in relative mortality in RA compared with the general population over the past 20 years. Consistent with these trends, the GBD 2010 study reported a decline in the age-standardized death rate from RA by 9.9% during the 1990–2010 period with a resulting estimated mortality rate at 0.8/100,000 in 2010 [11].

Cause specific mortality in rheumatoid arthritis, with a focus on cardiovascular disease

The significant contribution of comorbidities to the excess mortality in RA is increasingly recognized. The pattern of cause-specific mortality in RA seems to be relatively constant over time, with the major attributable causes of death in RA similar to that in the general population, including cardiovascular disease (CVD), respiratory diseases, hematologic disorders, infectious diseases, malignancies, genitourinary, and gastrointestinal disorders [13,14,21,22]. Of these disorders, CVD confers the greatest risk of mortality in RA.

Although not increasing, the relative cardiovascular mortality has not seemed to decline during the past decades. Integrating the findings published during the past 50 years, recent meta-analyses confirmed the substantial excess risk of cardiovascular death in patients with RA at 50–60%, with no apparent decrease in cardiovascular mortality up to the mid-2000s [23,24]. More recently published studies suggest that cardiovascular mortality in RA may be improving. The NOAR study was one of the first to report a trend towards decline in cardiovascular mortality from 8.78/1000 person years in a RA cohort who were first enrolled in the register in 1990–1994 to 7.07/1000 person years in those enrolled in 2000–2004 based on the 2010 ACR criteria for RA [20]. A trend towards decreasing CVD case fatality in RA patients has been suggested in a recent study comparing data from short-term prospective observations with cardiovascular mortality estimates reported in literature [25].

Concordantly, significant improvement in the overall cardiovascular mortality and coronary heart disease (CHD) mortality has been shown in Olmsted County, Minnesota for patients with incident RA in 2000–2007 compared to the previous decades [26]. Furthermore, there appears to be a significant improvement in the relative ten-year cardiovascular mortality including CHD mortality in patients with incident RA in 2000–2007 compared with the general population (Figure 1.3).

Taken together, these findings represent an important milestone in CVD management with potential implications on the role of inflammation and its control on CVD risk for both RA patients and the general population

[26]. Understanding the underlying nature for this improvement may aid in improving CVD risk management strategies.

In summary, recent studies suggest a significant improvement in overall mortality in RA patients over the last decades, likely reflecting major advances in RA disease management and inflammation control.

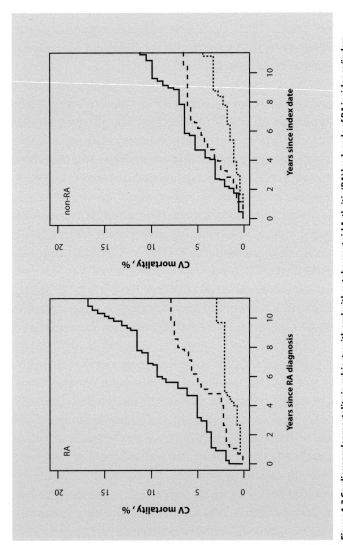

Figure 1.3 Cardiovascular mortality in subjects with and without rheumatoid Arthritis (RA) by decade of RA incidence/index: 1980–89 (solid line); 1990–99 (dashed line); 2000–07 (dotted line). Reproduced with permission from © John Wiley and Sons, 2015. All Rights Reserved. Myasoedova et al [26].

There is an emerging improvement in cardiovascular mortality with potential improvement in the relative cardiovascular mortality in RA compared with non-RA subjects. However, all-cause mortality in RA remains significantly elevated compared to the general population and no improvement in the overall mortality gap has been shown thus far. These data suggest unknown or unaddressed risk factors for mortality in RA compared with the general population. Several factors (including genes, autoimmune inflammatory burden, and increased comorbidity risk) may be potential determinants of the excess mortality in RA. More studies are needed to understand the underlying reasons for persistent mortality gap in RA.

Epidemiology and outcomes of cardiovascular disease in rheumatoid arthritis

Significantly increased risk of nearly all forms of CVD and excess in cardiovascular mortality in RA, which is not explained by traditional cardiovascular risk factors, has been reported in many epidemiological studies worldwide [23,27–29]. The role of RA as an independent risk factor for CVD, analogous to diabetes mellitus, has been increasingly recognized. The risk of development of fatal and non-fatal CVD events has been shown to be comparable in RA patients and in patients to diabetes while exceeding the general population estimates by approximately twofold, both in incident and prevalent CVD (Figure 1.4) [30–32].

Similar to diabetes, premature development of CVD, its silent nature, and unfavorable CVD outcomes have been repeatedly demonstrated as characteristic features of CVD in RA. The relative risk of CVD in RA has been shown to be highest in younger adults and in patients with RA without prior CVD [33]. The absolute CVD risk in RA patients appears to be similar to the non-RA subjects who are 5–10 years older, suggesting premature cardiovascular morbidity and mortality in RA [34].

Cardiovascular death in rheumatoid arthritis

Death from CVD is a leading cause of mortality in RA, accounting for approximately 40–50% of all deaths [21,35,36]. Increased risk of cardiovascular death is more pronounced in RA patients who are seropositive for RF and anti-citrullinated peptide antibody (ACPA) than in seronegative

RA patients [13,37–40]. The relative risk of death from CVD appears to be higher in younger patients who are under the age of 55 and in women [36]. However, the absolute difference in cardiovascular mortality rates may be highest in the older age groups [33].

There is some evidence to suggest that excess cardiovascular mortality evolves after, rather than before, the onset of RA. Indeed, in the meta-analysis by Avina-Zubieta et al, the weighted–pooled summary estimates of SMRs (meta-SMR) were higher in established RA cohorts than in inception cohorts (meta-SMR 1.56, 95% CI 1.45–1.68 and 1.19, 95% CI 0.86–1.68, respectively) [23]. This finding is in line with the results of the individual cohort studies from NOAR and the Dutch population, where excess cardiovascular mortality was detectable after 5–10 years after the onset of arthritis [14,36].

Coronary artery disease in rheumatoid arthritis
Coronary artery disease (CAD) is one of the major contributors to excess CVD risk and excess cardiovascular mortality in RA. The risk of CAD in RA

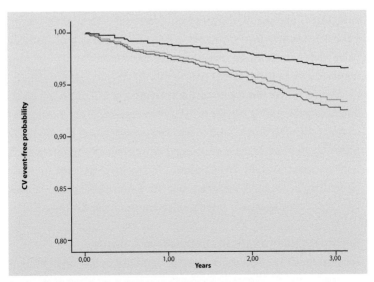

Figure 1.4 Cardiovascular event-free probability during three years among non-diabetic controls (black line), patients with Type 2 diabetes mellitus (light grey line), and non-diabetic patients with rheumatoid arthritis (dark grey line). Reproduced with permission from © John Wiley and Sons, 2009. All Rights Reserved. Peters et al [30].

patients is increased 1.5–2.0 fold compared with the general population [32,33,41]. A recent meta-analysis estimated a 68% increase in the risk of acute myocardial infarction (MI) in patients with RA compared with the general population (pooled relative risk [RR] 1.68; 95% CI 1.40–2.03), with significantly increased risk in both genders [42]. Increased coronary plaque burden even in RA patients without symptomatic CAD compared with non-RA subjects, and increased vulnerability of coronary plaques in RA compared with non-RA, may contribute to the increased risk of MI in RA versus the general population [43].

There is an ongoing discussion regarding the timing of onset of increased CVD risk in RA. Some studies suggest that the increase in CAD risk in RA may precede RA diagnosis. In the Olmsted County, Minnesota population, RA patients were significantly more likely to have been hospitalized with acute MI (odds ratio [OR] 3.17, 95% CI 1.16–8.68) or to have experienced unrecognized MIs (OR 5.86, 95% CI 1.29–26.64) during the two-year period preceding the diagnosis of RA compared with non-RA subjects [41].

Other studies have not found this association. No increase in the risk of CAD, angina, or heart failure (HF) prior to the onset of RA have been reported in two large Swedish cohorts of RA patients [44] although trends towards increase in risk could not be excluded. These authors reported that there was a rapid increase in the risk of MI during the first years following RA diagnosis (RR 1.6 (95% CI 1.4–1.9) compared to the general population of Sweden [45]. This latter observation is in line with the findings from the Olmsted County, Minnesota cohort where an approximately twofold increase in risk of unrecognized MIs (hazard ratio [HR] 2.13, 95% CI 1.13–4.03) and sudden cardiac deaths (HR 1.94, 95% CI 1.06–3.55) was detected after the RA incidence [41].

This increased risk is likely multifactorial, with inflammation being an important contributor, along with traditional CVD risk factors and anti-rheumatic medications, as discussed later in this book. However, some other less known contributors can be also considered. For instance, there is a growing body of literature on the disparity of CVD preventive measures in patients with RA versus those without RA.

Suboptimal treatment with antithrombotic medications in RA patients with prior MI or stroke has been shown in an international study on comorbidities in RA (COMORA) [46]. Some studies have reported that RA patients are less likely to undergo early coronary reperfusion, including thrombolysis and acute percutaneous coronary intervention [PCI]), and less likely to receive treatment with beta-blockers and lipid lowering medications after acute MI than non-RA subjects [47]. Lower likelihood of coronary artery bypass grafting (CABG) has been reported in patients with autoimmune inflammatory diseases including RA versus non-RA subjects [48]. These disparities in management of CAD have been suggested as a potential contributor to the increased risk for 30-day and 1-year mortality after MI in RA compared with the general population [48].

In contrast, other studies reported that RA patients were more likely to undergo thrombolysis or PCI after acute MI and had about 30% lower in-hospital mortality after acute MI compared with non-RA subjects [49,50]. However, concurrent with the previous studies, these authors reported lower likelihood of CABG in RA versus non-RA patients. No increase in operative or overall mortality after CABG was found in RA versus non-RA subjects [51].

A recent population-based cohort study in Olmsted County, Minnesota did not find any significant differences in MI treatment, or use of cardioprotective drugs in RA versus non-RA subjects, but reported poorer long-term outcomes including mortality (5-year mortality rates: 57% ± 6% in RA versus 36% ± 4% in non-RA; log-rank p=0.036; HR 1.47; 95% CI 1.04–2.08), and recurrent ischemia (HR 1.51; 95% CI 1.04–2.18) in RA patients compared with non-RA subjects [52]. More studies are needed to understand the role of health care disparities in CVD management and the impact they have on CVD outcomes in RA.

Heart failure in rheumatoid arthritis

There is compelling evidence of increased risk of HF in patients with RA [53,54]. Studies from Olmsted County, Minnesota have reported an 87% increase in the risk of incident HF in RA compared with the non-RA subjects during a 40-year observation (HR 1.87, 95% CI 1.47–2.39)

(Figure 1.5). This increase in risk was more pronounced in RA patients who were RF-positive rather than RF-negative [53]. The higher incidence of HF was found in all age groups of RA patients, although it tended to be higher in women than in men (RR 1.9, 95% CI 1.4–2.5 vs RR 1.3 95% CI 0.9–2.0, respectively).

Unlike in the general population where the large majority of HF cases are attributable to CAD, the excess risk of HF in RA is not explained by clinical CAD [53]. In fact, a recent study showed that the risk of development of HF after MI was similar among patients with and without RA (HR 1.30; 95% CI 0.81–2.10), although cumulative incidence of developing HF tended to be higher at 5 years after MI in patients with RA (57% ± 8%) than in the non-RA subjects (35% ± 4%, log-rank p=0.24) [52].

In a population-based incidence cohort of RA patients, Davis et al reported that a history of ischemic heart disease was less common in RA subjects with HF than in non-RA subjects with HF [28]. Furthermore, this study highlighted several other important differentiating features of HF in RA. These included increased prevalence of HF with preserved

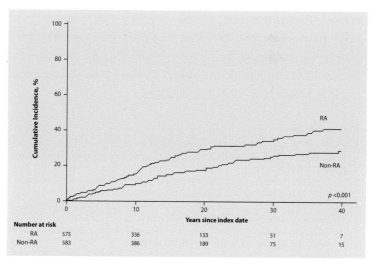

Figure 1.5 Cumulative incidence of heart failure in rheumatoid arthritis versus non-rheumatoid arthritis subjects. Reproduced with permission from © John Wiley and Sons, 2005. All Rights Reserved. Nicola et al [53].

ejection fraction (HFPEF), lack of typical HF symptoms, lower likelihood of undergoing echocardiography, and a 1.9-fold increased mortality in the year following HF (HR 1.89, 95% CI 1.26–2.84) in RA versus non-RA subjects. The increased prevalence of HFPEF in RA likely represents left ventricular (LV) diastolic dysfunction, suggesting that mechanisms of HF in RA differ from those in the general population and may be related to systemic inflammation. Higher RA disease activity has been linked to increased LV relative wall thickness, a strong predictor of adverse cardiovascular outcomes [55]. This suggests potential benefits of RA disease control for prevention of prognostically unfavorable changes in myocardial structure and function, with expectations for improved cardiovascular outcomes in RA.

In summary, there is convincing evidence of substantially increased burden of nearly all forms of CVD and resulting increase in cardiovascular mortality in RA compared with the general population. CAD and HF are among the major contributors of increased cardiovascular morbidity in RA, consistently associated with adverse CVD outcomes. A peculiar pattern of CVD in RA including its premature onset, atypical clinical features, rapid progression, increased risk of adverse CVD outcomes, and perhaps some inequities in CVD management put patients with RA at a major disadvantage for CVD control compared with the general population. Similar to diabetes, RA has been postulated as an independent risk factor for CVD suggesting that adequate control of RA disease activity would be beneficial for CVD risk reduction.

References

1   Alamanos Y, Voulgari PV, Drosos AA. Incidence and prevalence of rheumatoid arthritis, based on the 1987 American College of Rheumatology criteria: a systematic review. *Semin Arthritis Rheum*. 2006;36:182-188.
2   Hochberg MC. Changes in the incidence and prevalence of rheumatoid arthritis in England and Wales, 1970-1982. *Semin Arthritis Rheum*. 1990;19:294-302.
3   Kaipiainen-Seppanen O, Aho K, Isomaki H, Laakso M. Incidence of rheumatoid arthritis in Finland during 1980-1990. *Ann Rheum Dis*. 1996;55:608-611.
4   Gabriel SE, Crowson CS, O'Fallon WM. The epidemiology of rheumatoid arthritis in Rochester, Minnesota, 1955-1985. *Arthritis Rheum*. 1999;42:415-420.
5   Shichikawa K, Inoue K, Hirota S, et al. Changes in the incidence and prevalence of rheumatoid arthritis in Kamitonda, Wakayama, Japan, 1965-1996. *Ann Rheum Dis*. 1999;58:751-756.
6   Doran MF, Pond GR, Crowson CS, O'Fallon WM, Gabriel SE. Trends in incidence and mortality in rheumatoid arthritis in Rochester, Minnesota, over a forty-year period. *Arthritis Rheum*. 2002;46:625-631.

7   Kaipiainen-Seppanen O, Kautiainen H. Declining trend in the incidence of rheumatoid factor-positive rheumatoid arthritis in Finland 1980-2000. *J Rheumatol*. 2006;33:2132-2138.

8   Jacobsson LT, Hanson RL, Knowler WC, et al. Decreasing incidence and prevalence of rheumatoid arthritis in Pima Indians over a twenty-five-year period. *Arthritis Rheum*. 1994;37:1158-1165.

9   Akushevich I, Kravchenko J, Ukraintseva S, Arbeev K, Yashin AI. Time trends of incidence of age-associated diseases in the US elderly population: Medicare-based analysis. *Age Ageing*. 2013;42:494-500.

10   Myasoedova E, Crowson CS, Kremers HM, Therneau TM, Gabriel SE. Is the incidence of rheumatoid arthritis rising?: results from Olmsted County, Minnesota, 1955-2007. *Arthritis Rheum*. 2010;62:1576-1582.

11   Cross M, Smith E, Hoy D, et al. The global burden of rheumatoid arthritis: estimates from the global burden of disease 2010 study. *Ann Rheum Dis*. 2014;73:1316-1322.

12   Gonzalez A, Maradit Kremers H, Crowson CS, et al. The widening mortality gap between rheumatoid arthritis patients and the general population. *Arthritis Rheum*. 2007;56:3583-3587.

13   Gonzalez A, Icen M, Kremers HM, et al. Mortality trends in rheumatoid arthritis: the role of rheumatoid factor. *J Rheumatol*. 2008;35:1009-1014.

14   Radovits BJ, Fransen J, Al Shamma S, Eijsbouts AM, van Riel PL, Laan RF. Excess mortality emerges after 10 years in an inception cohort of early rheumatoid arthritis. *Arthritis Care Res (Hoboken)*. 2010;62:362-370.

15   Ziade N, Jougla E, Coste J. Population-level influence of rheumatoid arthritis on mortality and recent trends: a multiple cause-of-death analysis in France, 1970-2002. *J Rheumatol*. 2008;35:1950-1957.

16   Bergstrom U, Jacobsson LT, Turesson C. Cardiovascular morbidity and mortality remain similar in two cohorts of patients with long-standing rheumatoid arthritis seen in 1978 and 1995 in Malmo, Sweden. *Rheumatology (Oxford)*. 2009;48:1600-1605.

17   Dadoun S, Zeboulon-Ktorza N, Combescure C, et al. Mortality in rheumatoid arthritis over the last fifty years: systematic review and meta-analysis. *Joint Bone Spine*. 2013;80:29-33.

18   Crowson CS, Myasoedova E, Matteson EL, Kremers HM, Therneau TM, Gabriel SE. Has survival improved in patients recently diagnosed with rheumatoid arthritis? *Arthritis Rheum*. 2009;60:1172.

19   Widdifield J, Bernatsky S, Paterson JM, et al. Trends in excess mortality among patients with rheumatoid arthritis in Ontario, Canada. *Arthritis Care Res (Hoboken)*. 2015;67:1047-1053.

20   Humphreys JH, Warner A, Chipping J, et al. Mortality trends in patients with early rheumatoid arthritis over 20 years: results from the Norfolk Arthritis Register. *Arthritis Care Res (Hoboken)*. 2014;66:1296-1301.

21   Sokka T, Abelson B, Pincus T. Mortality in rheumatoid arthritis: 2008 update. *Clin Exp Rheumatol*. 2008;26:S35-S61.

22   England BR, Sayles H, Michaud K, et al. Cause-specific mortality in US veteran men with rheumatoid arthritis. *Arthritis Care Res (Hoboken)*. 20156;68:35-45.

23   Avina-Zubieta JA, Choi HK, Sadatsafavi M, Etminan M, Esdaile JM, Lacaille D. Risk of cardiovascular mortality in patients with rheumatoid arthritis: a meta-analysis of observational studies. *Arthritis Rheum*. 2008;59:1690-1697.

24   Meune C, Touze E, Trinquart L, Allanore Y. Trends in cardiovascular mortality in patients with rheumatoid arthritis over 50 years: a systematic review and meta-analysis of cohort studies. *Rheumatology (Oxford)*. 2009;48:1309-1313.

25   Meek IL, Vonkeman HE, van de Laar MA. Cardiovascular case fatality in rheumatoid arthritis is decreasing; first prospective analysis of a current low disease activity rheumatoid arthritis cohort and review of the literature. *BMC Musculoskelet Disord*. 2014;15:142.

26   Myasoedova E CC, Matteson EL, Davis JM III, Therneau TM, Gabriel SE. Decreased cardiovascular mortality in patients with incident rheumatoid arthritis (RA) in recent years: dawn of a new era in cardiovascualar disease in RA? *Arthritis Rheumatol*. 2015;67.

27 Wolfe F, Michaud K. The risk of myocardial infarction and pharmacologic and nonpharmacologic myocardial infarction predictors in rheumatoid arthritis: a cohort and nested case-control analysis. *Arthritis Rheum*. 2008;58:2612-2621.

28 Davis JM, 3rd, Roger VL, Crowson CS, Kremers HM, Therneau TM, Gabriel SE. The presentation and outcome of heart failure in patients with rheumatoid arthritis differs from that in the general population. *Arthritis Rheum*. 2008;58:2603-2611.

29 Masuda H, Miyazaki T, Shimada K, et al. Disease duration and severity impacts on long-term cardiovascular events in Japanese patients with rheumatoid arthritis. *J Cardiol*. 2014;64: 366-370.

30 Peters MJ, van Halm VP, Voskuyl AE, et al. Does rheumatoid arthritis equal diabetes mellitus as an independent risk factor for cardiovascular disease? A prospective study. *Arthritis Rheum*. 2009;61:1571-1579.

31 van Halm VP, Peters MJ, Voskuyl AE, et al. Rheumatoid arthritis versus diabetes as a risk factor for cardiovascular disease: a cross-sectional study, the CARRE Investigation. *Ann Rheum Dis*. 2009;68:1395-1400.

32 Lindhardsen J, Ahlehoff O, Gislason GH, et al. The risk of myocardial infarction in rheumatoid arthritis and diabetes mellitus: a Danish nationwide cohort study. *Ann Rheum Dis*. 2011;70:929-934.

33 Solomon DH, Goodson NJ, Katz JN, et al. Patterns of cardiovascular risk in rheumatoid arthritis. *Ann Rheum Dis*. 2006;65:1608-1612.

34 Kremers HM, Crowson CS, Therneau TM, Roger VL, Gabriel SE. High ten-year risk of cardiovascular disease in newly diagnosed rheumatoid arthritis patients: a population-based cohort study. *Arthritis Rheum*. 2008;58:2268-2274.

35 Wallberg-Jonsson S, Ohman ML, Dahlqvist SR. Cardiovascular morbidity and mortality in patients with seropositive rheumatoid arthritis in Northern Sweden. *J Rheumatol*. 1997;24:445-451.

36 Naz SM, Farragher TM, Bunn DK, Symmons DP, Bruce IN. The influence of age at symptom onset and length of followup on mortality in patients with recent-onset inflammatory polyarthritis. *Arthritis Rheum*. 2008;58:985-989.

37 Goodson NJ, Wiles NJ, Lunt M, Barrett EM, Silman AJ, Symmons DP. Mortality in early inflammatory polyarthritis: cardiovascular mortality is increased in seropositive patients. *Arthritis Rheum*. 2002;46:2010-2019.

38 Goodson NJ, Symmons DP, Scott DG, Bunn D, Lunt M, Silman AJ. Baseline levels of C-reactive protein and prediction of death from cardiovascular disease in patients with inflammatory polyarthritis: a ten-year followup study of a primary care-based inception cohort. *Arthritis Rheum*. 2005;52:2293-2299.

39 Farragher TM, Goodson NJ, Naseem H, et al. Association of the HLA-DRB1 gene with premature death, particularly from cardiovascular disease, in patients with rheumatoid arthritis and inflammatory polyarthritis. *Arthritis Rheum*. 2008;58:359-369.

40 Ajeganova S, Andersson ML, Frostegard J, Hafstrom I. Disease factors in early rheumatoid arthritis are associated with differential risks for cardiovascular events and mortality depending on age at onset: a 10-year observational cohort study. *J Rheumatol*. 2013;40: 1958-1966.

41 Maradit-Kremers H, Crowson CS, Nicola PJ, et al. Increased unrecognized coronary heart disease and sudden deaths in rheumatoid arthritis: a population-based cohort study. *Arthritis Rheum*. 2005;52:402-411.

42 Avina-Zubieta JA, Thomas J, Sadatsafavi M, Lehman AJ, Lacaille D. Risk of incident cardiovascular events in patients with rheumatoid arthritis: a meta-analysis of observational studies. *Ann Rheum Dis*. 2012;71:1524-1529.

43 Karpouzas GA, Malpeso J, Choi TY, Li D, Munoz S, Budoff MJ. Prevalence, extent and composition of coronary plaque in patients with rheumatoid arthritis without symptoms or prior diagnosis of coronary artery disease. *Ann Rheum Dis*. 2014;73:1797-1804.

44 Holmqvist ME, Wedren S, Jacobsson LT, et al. No increased occurrence of ischemic heart disease prior to the onset of rheumatoid arthritis: results from two Swedish population-based rheumatoid arthritis cohorts. *Arthritis Rheum*. 2009;60:2861-2869.

45 Holmqvist ME, Wedren S, Jacobsson LT, et al. Rapid increase in myocardial infarction risk following diagnosis of rheumatoid arthritis amongst patients diagnosed between 1995 and 2006. *J Intern Med*. 2010;268:578-585.

46 Dougados M, Soubrier M, Antunez A, et al. Prevalence of comorbidities in rheumatoid arthritis and evaluation of their monitoring: results of an international, cross-sectional study (COMORA). *Ann Rheum Dis*. 2014;73:62-68.

47 Van Doornum S, Brand C, Sundararajan V, Ajani AE, Wicks IP. Rheumatoid arthritis patients receive less frequent acute reperfusion and secondary prevention therapy after myocardial infarction compared with the general population. *Arthritis Res Ther*. 2010;12:R183.

48 Van Doornum S, Bohensky M, Tacey MA, Brand CA, Sundararajan V, Wicks IP. Increased 30-day and 1-year mortality rates and lower coronary revascularisation rates following acute myocardial infarction in patients with autoimmune rheumatic disease. *Arthritis Res Ther*. 2015;17:38.

49 Francis ML, Varghese JJ, Mathew JM, Koneru S, Scaife SL, Zahnd WE. Outcomes in patients with rheumatoid arthritis and myocardial infarction. *Am J Med*. 2010;123:922-928.

50 Varghese JJ, Koneru S, Scaife SL, Zahnd WE, Francis ML. Mortality after coronary artery revascularization of patients with rheumatoid arthritis. *J Thorac Cardiovasc Surg*. 2010;140:91-96.

51 Lai CH, Lai WW, Chiou MJ, Tsai LM, Wen JS, Li CY. Outcomes of coronary artery bypass grafting in patients with inflammatory rheumatic diseases: an 11-year nationwide cohort study. *J Thorac Cardiovasc Surg*. 2015;149:859-866.

52 McCoy SS, Crowson CS, Maradit-Kremers H, et al. Longterm outcomes and treatment after myocardial infarction in patients with rheumatoid arthritis. *J Rheumatol*. 2013;40:605-610.

53 Nicola PJ, Maradit-Kremers H, Roger VL, et al. The risk of congestive heart failure in rheumatoid arthritis: a population-based study over 46 years. *Arthritis Rheum*. 2005;52:412-420.

54 Wolfe F, Michaud K. Heart failure in rheumatoid arthritis: rates, predictors, and the effect of anti-tumor necrosis factor therapy. *Am J Med*. 2004;116:305-311.

55 Midtbo H, Gerdts E, Kvien TK, et al. Disease activity and left ventricular structure in patients with rheumatoid arthritis. *Rheumatology (Oxford)*. 2015;54:511-519.

Chapter 2

Non-atherosclerotic cardiac manifestations of rheumatoid arthritis

Rekha Mankad, Carolyn A Ball, Elena Myasoedova, and
Eric L Matteson

Pericardial diseases

First clearly described by Charcot in the 19th century, pericardial disease
has been regarded as the most common cardiac manifestation of rheumatoid arthritis (RA). Pericarditis has been shown to affect about one-
third of RA patients, with some variations in prevalence from 30 to 50%
depending on the diagnostic method (ie, echocardiography versus post-
mortem examination) and the calendar period under study [1–4]. While
in most cases pericarditis develops after the onset of RA, some studies
have demonstrated that it can precede RA diagnosis and may be the first
manifestation of RA disease activity. A recent systematic review and
meta-analysis of case-control studies from 1975 through 2010 reported
that the risk of developing pericardial effusion was tenfold higher in
patients with RA compared with non-RA subjects (odds ratio [OR] 10.7;
95% confidence interval [CI] 5.0–23.0) [2].

Pericardial disease in RA is frequently asymptomatic. Only a minority
of patients (<10%), most commonly males, with severe rheumatoid factor
(RF)-positive and often with nodular RA, develop clinical pericarditis
[1,5]. The annual incidence of clinically manifest pericarditis in RA has

© Springer International Publishing Switzerland 2017
A.G. Semb (ed.), *Handbook of Cardiovascular Disease Management
in Rheumatoid Arthritis*, DOI 10.1007/978-3-319-26782-1_2

been found to be 0.34% in females and 0.44% in males [5]. The majority of symptomatic patients present with acute pericarditis [3]. Progression from exudative to constrictive pericarditis has been described in up to one-fourth of patients [6]. Similar to rheumatoid pleural effusions, pericardial effusions in patients with RA are commonly sterile, with variable leukocyte counts, high protein levels, decreased complement and glucose levels, and presence of RF and immune complexes [2,4,5]. Although rare, cholesterol pericarditis presenting as pericardial effusion with high cholesterol content, and in some cases with progression to constrictive pericarditis, has been described in patients with RA [7]. Symptomatic pericarditis is associated with increased mortality in patients with RA, predominantly in the first year of follow-up [3,8]. The highest mortality rates were observed in RA patients with constrictive and rapidly progressive pericarditis [8]. Chronic pericardial disease has been described in patients with severe long-standing RA, some of them initially presenting with cardiac tamponade requiring urgent surgical management [2,3].

More recently, there has been emerging evidence of the association between treatment with biologic disease-modifying antirheumatic drugs (bDMARDs) and development of pericarditis. While biologic response modifiers (BRM) generally appear to be associated with better control of articular and some extra-articular manifestations of RA including vasculitis, several reports have described development of acute and/or recurrent pericarditis, occasionally with tamponade, in patients treated with tumor necrosis factor (TNF) inhibitors, requiring discontinuation of anti-TNF treatment and often surgical management (ie, pericardiectomy, pericardial window, or drain) [9]. Most of these cases have been associated with a non-infective pericardial effusion, which was thought to be due to a paradoxical RA flare in the setting of anti-TNF therapy [9]. However, cases of infective pericarditis with purulent pericardial effusion in RA patients on anti-TNF inhibitors or the B-lymphocyte inhibitor rituximab, with or without combination therapy with traditional disease modifying anti rheumatic drugs (DMARDs), have also been described [10,11]. These patients required prolonged systemic antibiotic therapy.

Diagnosis

Pericardial disease is typically diagnosed with echocardiography. Transthoracic echocardiography (TTE) is performed when there are symptoms or signs suggestive of pericarditis, pericardial effusion, or constrictive pericarditis. A small pericardial effusion is the most common finding. TTE is frequently used as the initial diagnostic tool used to establish the diagnosis of constrictive pericarditis; however, alternative imaging may be required to help aid in the diagnosis. Cardiac magnetic resonance (CMR) imaging is able to diagnose pericardial effusions, pericardial thickening (Figure 2.1), and pericarditis, using special techniques that identify inflammation (Figure 2.2A and B).

Treatment

Asymptomatic pericardial effusions can be self-limiting, particularly when the effusion is small. Mild symptomatic pericarditis usually responds well to treatment with aspirin or non-steroidal anti-inflammatory drugs (NSAIDs), primarily ibuprofen [12]. Glucocorticoid therapy may be used

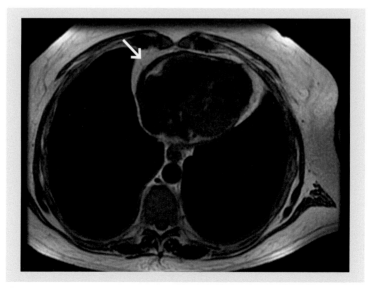

Figure 2.1 Magnetic resonance imaging in a patient with rheumatoid arthritis. Axial double inversion recovery sequence demonstrates pericardial thickening, measuring 6 mm (arrow). Courtesy of Dr Crystal Bonnichsen, Division of Cardiovascular Diseases, Mayo Clinic, Rochester, Minnesota.

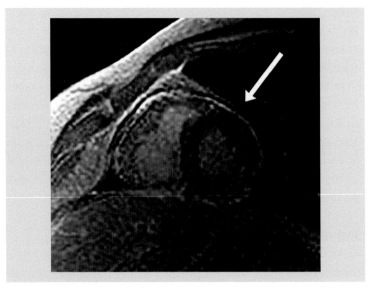

Figure 2.2 (A) Short axis delayed enhancement image shows bright enhancement of the pericardium (arrows) consistent with pericardial inflammation.

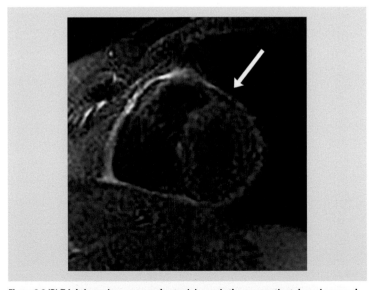

Figure 2.2 (B) Triple inversion recovery short axis image in the same patient shows increased signal in the pericardium (arrow), which indicates pericardial edema and active inflammation. **Courtesy of Dr Philip Araoz, Department of Radiology, Mayo Clinic, Rochester, Minnesota.**

in more severe disease, in cases of contraindications to aspirin/NSAIDs, or failure of one or more NSAIDs. The use of low-to-moderate doses of glucocorticoids is recommended (ie, prednisone 0.2–0.5 mg/kg/day). Treatment with either NSAIDs or glucocorticoids should continue until complete resolution of symptoms and normalization of inflammatory marker levels. Glucocorticoids should be tapered off slowly, after remission has been achieved. Colchicine can be used in addition to aspirin, NSAIDs, or glucocorticoids to improve disease control and decrease the rate of recurrence. There is weaker evidence to support the use of other treatment regimens especially in patients with recurrent or refractory disease, including azathioprine and other immunosuppressive drugs, intravenous immunoglobulin, or other bDMARDS such as interleukin 1 (IL-1) inhibitors for example, anakinra [13]. The use of these agents should be limited to cases where conventional medications have failed to produce adequate disease control [12].

While most cases of RA-related pericarditis can be effectively managed with medications, some severe cases associated with cardiac tamponade, and hemodynamically significant pericardial effusion, constrictive or effusive-constrictive physiology, and chronic or treatment-refractory pericarditis may require surgical management. Invasive techniques include pericardiocentesis, pericardiectomy, or pericardiotomy ('window' pericardiectomy) [12].

Myocardial diseases

Compared with pericardial disease, myocardial involvement in RA is less common. Post-mortem studies report findings consistent with either diffuse or focal myocarditis in 11–20% patients with RA [14,15]. However, most RA patients with myocarditis are clinically asymptomatic and the disease follows a self-limiting course. Symptomatic myocarditis is rare and is usually associated with active articular disease and other extra articular disease manifestations of RA (ExRA). In these more severe, clinically manifest cases, complications such as secondary cardiomyopathy and resulting heart failure (HF) as well as cardiac arrhythmias and conduction abnormalities can occur [16,17].

The prevalence of RA-associated cardiomyopathy is not well understood and large cohort studies on the subject are lacking. A small case series of 30 patients with RA suggested a 37% prevalence of cardiomyopathy based on echocardiography studies [18]. Both ischemic and secondary non-ischemic cardiomyopathies resulting from either non-specific or granulomatous myocarditis or anti-rheumatic medication use, such as glucocorticoids and antimalarial medication, have been described in RA [4].

Myocarditis in RA follows one of the two histological patterns:

1. a granulomatous form that is considered specific for RA, with morphological features typical for subcutaneous RA nodules and predilection for the myocardium of the left ventricle (LV); and

2. a non-specific form that is also observed in other disorders and is morphologically characterized by interstitial infiltration with lymphocytes, plasma cells, and histiocytes [14].

Imaging and myocardial disease

Among imaging studies, echocardiography has been commonly used to assess the LV ejection fraction (EF) in patients with concern for myocardial involvement; however this technique is not able to detect myocardial inflammation and thus appears to be unsuitable for detection of myocarditis. CMR imaging has been evolving as a useful non-invasive modality for early diagnosis of myocardial tissue abnormalities providing results similar to myocardial biopsy [19].

A few characteristic imaging features of myocardial involvement have been suggested in patients without cardiovascular symptoms but with active RA based on standardized CMR study. These include an increased T2-weighted edema ratio (ER) score suggesting myocardial tissue edema, myocardial wall thinning, and cavity dilatation, with reduced global EF and globally raised late gadolinium enhancement (LGE) scores, potentially reflecting diffuse myocardial fibrosis resulting from microvascular disease, macrovascular CAD, and chronic myocardial inflammation [20]. With the introduction of higher resolution techniques for improved myocardial imaging, such as 3- and 7-Tesla scanners, the diagnostic possibilities for myocardial imaging may expand significantly in the near future, with corresponding opportunities for earlier recognition and timely management of myocardial involvement in RA [19].

Treatment

Due to the rare occurrence of rheumatoid myocarditis, optimal treatment has not been established and evidence-based guidelines on management of myocarditis in RA are lacking. Conventional cardiovascular treatment aimed at support of LV function in conjunction with aggressive anti-inflammatory therapy and treatment with DMARDs theoretically should be beneficial. High-dose glucocorticoid therapy has been associated with resolution of imaging abnormalities, normalization of LV function and resolution of HF symptoms in a patient with rheumatoid vasculitis and myocardial involvement [21]. The resolution of conduction abnormalities associated with myocarditis in RA may also occur when the underlying RA disease is well-controlled [22].

Azathioprine and cyclophosphamide can be used in RA patients who did not respond to high-dose glucocorticoids. The role of bDMARDs (particularly anti-TNF agents) in the management of rheumatoid myocarditis remains uncertain, which is in part due to concerns for potential harm associated with anti-TNF agents use in advanced HF [23].

Antimalarial agents and cardiomyopathy

Over the past two decades there has been growing evidence of the association between the use of antimalarial agents, primarily chloroquine and hydroxychloroquine, and myocardial toxicity, clinically manifesting as HF in the setting of restrictive or dilated cardiomyopathy and/or conduction abnormalities in RA patients [24]. The exact mechanism of the cardiomyopathy associated with the use of antimalarials remains unclear but may involve lysosomal changes and accumulation of glycogen and phospholipids resulting in a vacuolar type of myopathy [24] including enlarged and vacuolated cells on light microscopy. Electron microscopy processing shows cytoplasmic granules with curvilinear and myelin-like configurations ('myeloid bodies'), thought to be abnormal lysosomes, pathognomonic to antimalarial cardiotoxicity [24,25]. In the absence of specific treatment, prognosis in antimalarial cardiotoxicity ranges from partial or complete recovery of cardiac function with early recognition of antimalarial toxicity and timely withdrawal of the offending drug to heart transplantation or death in unrecognized cases.

Cardiac amyloidosis

Cardiac amyloidosis is a rare manifestation of systemic RA-associated amyloid A (AA)-amyloidosis. Exact estimates of incidence and prevalence of cardiac amyloidosis are lacking, which is in part due to unrecognized disease. Myocardial infiltration with amyloid and progressive myocardial fibrotic changes results in myocardial hypertrophy, impairment of systolic and diastolic function in the setting of restrictive cardiomyopathy, and subsequent unfavorable cardiovascular outcomes and increased mortality [19].

While histological diagnosis is a gold standard for the diagnosis of cardiac amyloidosis, its use is limited due to the invasive nature of myocardial biopsy. Increased echogenicity of the myocardium with a granular or 'sparkling' appearance on TTE has been associated with a diagnosis of cardiac amyloidosis. However, these myocardial characteristics have been found in other causes of LV hypertrophy, and despite high specificity (up to 80%) the sensitivity of this pattern of echocardiographic findings for diagnosis of cardiac amyloid has been generally low (about 30%) [26,27]. Several studies have demonstrated a pattern of LGE on CMR imaging, suggestive of cardiac amyloid depositions, in patients with systemic amyloidosis [28]. Thus, newer modalities of CMR may be promising in means of identifying early phenotypical features of cardiac amyloidosis.

The prognosis of patients with cardiac amyloidosis is generally poor due to associated progressive HF. The use of cytotoxic drugs and bDMARDs can help to temporarily improve cardiac function [29,30]. However, progressive organ failure can occur despite aggressive treatment.

Non-atherosclerotic coronary artery disease

In addition to atherosclerotic disease, myocardial ischemia can occur in RA patients secondary to vasculitis. Coronary vasculitis is often associated with the rheumatologic vasculitides but can also occur in RA [31]. The term rheumatoid vasculitis (RV) has been coined to refer to the development of inflammation in the wall of the blood vessels in patients with RA. Typically, this process involves the medium-sized muscular arteries through to the smaller arterioles or post-capillary venules. Rheumatoid vasculitis tends to occur in those patients with longer stand-ing, erosive disease and manifests in those patients who have had RA for more than 10 years. An early autopsy study places the incidence of epicardial vasculitis at 20%. In this study, the affected vessels identified as involving vasculitis were in various stages of healing, and of variable clinical significance [31,32]. Vasculitis of the epicardial arteries can lead to ischemia similar to epicardial atherosclerotic disease. Moreover, vasculitis of the small intramural cardiac vessels can lead to myocardial ischemia, and vasculitis of the vaso-vasorum can result in epicardial vessel dysfunction [32]. Vasculitis can also promote the development of atherosclerotic disease in affected vessels [33]. Overall, rheumatoid vasculitis has ranging levels of severity and clinical manifestations but can be associated with greater morbidity and mortality than the RA itself.

Arrhythmias

Arrhythmias are a significant component of the cardiac manifestations of RA and are an area of ongoing research. There is an increased risk of sudden cardiac death in patients with RA compared with the non-RA cohort [34]. Arrhythmias in RA patients may be due to the RA process itself or, more commonly, due to ischemic disease, heart failure, or amyloid deposition.

Atrial arrhythmias

The role of RA in the development of atrial fibrillation (AF) is an area of debate. Although population-based studies have conflicting attribut-able risk of AF to RA, there are several risk factors for AF that are more common in the RA population. In the general population there is an increased risk of the development, recurrence, and persistence of atrial fibrillation in patients with underlying inflammation. This has been spe-cifically demonstrated in patients with elevated TNF-alpha, IL-2, IL-6, and C-reactive protein (CRP) [35,36]. Based on these findings it would seem likely that patients with RA, particularly untreated or undertreated

RA, would have an increased risk of developing AF. Patients with RA have increased p-wave dispersion (PWD) [37]. PWD is a measure of the difference of p wave duration on a surface electrocardiogram and represents inhomogeneous conduction through the atria. In the non-RA cohort, increased PWD is a predictor of AF [38]. In the RA population, PWD correlates with CRP levels, suggesting increased inflammation may increase a patient's risk of AF [37]. However, in the RA population PWD has not been demonstrated to correlate with the prevalence of AF. In the general population, there is evidence that increased inflammatory markers are associated with an increased risk of AF, and that controlling inflammation can reduce the incidence [34]. Again, this has not been demonstrated in the RA population.

There have been two major studies examining the prevalence of AF in patients with RA. A Danish study found an overall incidence of AF that was 40% higher in the RA cohort than in the general population [39]. A health claim database study and another population based study from the United States found no increase in incidence of AF in patients with RA after adjusting for potential confounders [40,41].

Conduction system disease

In a review of electrocardiograms (ECGs) of patients with RA, the RA group had slightly longer PR intervals than their non-RA peers but the mean PR intervals in both groups were within normal limits [42]. In the same study there was a low prevalence of low degree atrioventricular (AV) blocks in the RA cohort. Most of the AV blocks in RA patients were third degree blocks [22]. Complete AV nodal blocks in RA patients have been associated with AV nodal infiltration by rheumatoid nodules, mononuclear cells, extension of inflammatory lesions from valvular involvement, and amyloid deposition [4,22]. Medications for RA have also been implicated in the development of complete heart block, including chloroquine.

Beyond the atrioventricular node, rheumatoid nodules can contribute to additional conduction system disease [4]. However, treating the underlying RA disease process with immunosuppressive therapies has not been shown to treat the arrhythmias due to rheumatoid nodules. In addition, pro-inflammatory cytokines, particularly TNF-alpha, may prolong myocyte action potential, predisposing to re-entrant ventricular arrhythmias [34].

Fibrosis secondary to RA can involve the conduction system, resulting in arrhythmias. Additionally, antibodies to cardiac conducting tissue, including Purkinje cells, can contribute to arrhythmia development [22].

Ventricular arrhythmias

Patients with RA are twice as likely to experience sudden cardiac death (SCD) as those without RA, even after adjusting for a history of myocardial infarction [43]. The mechanism of this increased incidence of SCD in RA patients remains unclear, but there is evidence that it may be due to the role of systemic inflammation in RA beyond atherosclerotic disease as well as autonomic dysfunction in RA patients [34].

Systemic inflammation, particularly inflammation within ventricular tissues, may lead to a delay in ventricular repolarization. This is manifest as an increased QT interval on an ECG, which is indeed seen more commonly in RA patients. One study found that after the diagnosis of RA, patients were more likely to develop prolonged heart rate corrected QT interval (QTc) than patients who were not diagnosed with RA [44]. Similarly, elevated CRP and positive anti-CCP are associated with prolonged QTc. Erythrocyte sedimentation rate (ESR) and RF have also been shown to trend positively toward prolonged QTc [45]. Pro-inflammatory cytokines, particularly TNF-alpha, may prolong myocyte action potential, predisposing to re-entrant ventricular arrhythmias, although this has not been specifically demonstrated [34]. Interestingly, patients with RA and prolonged QTc have increased all-cause mortality relative to their RA peers without prolonged QTc, but no difference in cardiovascular mortality compared to their RA peers [44,44]. This discrepancy suggests there may be another mechanism leading to increased ventricular arrhythmias and sudden cardiac death in the RA population.

Additional research into the mechanism for increased sudden cardiac death in patients with RA focuses on increased sympathetic tone in RA patients [34]. Heart rate variability is often used as a marker of sympathetic drive and parasympathetic suppression, with decreased heart rate variability indicating increased sympathetic drive. RA patients demonstrate decreased heart rate variability compared with non-RA peers [46]. In one study, women with RA were found to have a higher resting heart rate compared with their non-RA peers, suggesting decreased vagal tone as well as decreased heart rate variability, further pointing to a higher sympathetic drive. The increased sympathetic drive may be due to the so-called 'inflammatory reflex' in which pro-inflammatory cytokines target the autonomic centers of the brain. This, in turn, increases sympathetic drive to ultimately inhibit cytokine production and self-regulate inflammation [46]. There are currently no anti-arrhythmic therapies that specifically address arrhythmias in the RA population. Treatment of arrhythmia in a patient with RA should focus on the underlying rhythm disturbance [22].

Valvular heart disease

Valvular heart disease (VHD) is a known extra-articular complication of RA [2]. However, there is much uncertainty regarding the prevalence and pathophysiology of VHD in RA. There are several challenges to studying valve disease in RA patients. The majority of VHD in RA patients is asymptomatic, making prevalence studies difficult to conduct [2,18]. The prevalence of VHD in RA is significantly higher in autopsy studies than in echocardiographic studies. Additionally, as cardiac imaging technology advances, the ability to characterize subclinical valve disease will increase. VHD in RA presents in multiple forms, and has an inconsistent relationship with a systemic inflammatory disease course, making it difficult to select patients for studies.

Mechanisms of valvular heart disease

There are three major categories of valve destruction in RA: fibrosis, calcification, and granuloma formation. All three pathologies can be found on any of the cardiac valves, however, RA VHD is significantly more common on the left-sided valves, and most studies suggest that the mitral valve is most commonly affected.

Valvular fibrosis

Valve thickening is the most commonly described valvular pathology in RA. Autopsy and surgical pathology studies find thickening and fibrosis of each of the cardiac valves in RA patients, although the mitral valve is most commonly involved (Figure 2.3 and 2.4). Acute or recurrent valvulitis can cause thickening of the valve and is the result of infiltration of the valve tissue with plasma cells, histiocytes, lymphocytes, and eosinophils producing valve fibrosis, and, ultimately, valve retraction [47]. Echocardiographic studies have demonstrated a similar frequency of focal and diffuse involvement of valvulitis in patients with RA. Focal valvulitis affects the base, mid, and tip portions of the valves equally, and less commonly affects the mitral annulus or chordae tendineae. Valvular fibrosis in RA patients is similar to natural valve aging described in the general population, and, indeed, some patients with RA may demonstrate both RA-driven valvulitis in addition to aging or atherosclerotic valve fibrosis. No relationship has been identified between the presentation of valve fibrosis and the duration of inflammatory disease. Rheumatoid aortitis (extremely rare in the present day) can occur and may lead to

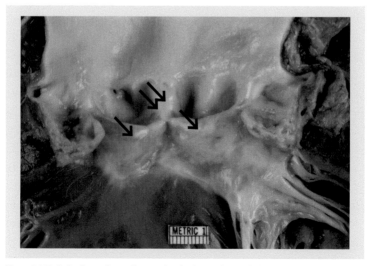

Figure 2.3 Pathologic specimen of an aortic valve in a patient with rheumatoid arthritis. Valve thickening (single arrow), and commissural fusion (double arrow). Courtesy of Dr William Edwards, Department of Laboratory Medicine and Pathology, Mayo Clinic, Rochester, Minnesota.

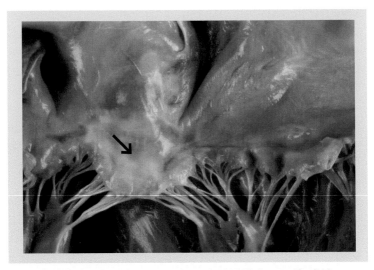

Figure 2.4 Pathologic specimen of a mitral valve in a patient with rheumatoid arthritis.
Marked thickening of the anterior leaflet of the mitral valve (arrow). Courtesy of Dr William Edwards, Department of Laboratory Medicine and Pathology, Mayo Clinic, Rochester, Minnesota.

aortic valve regurgitation (along with aortic aneurysms). Typically, this has been reported post-mortem [48]. Treatment with high-dose glucocorticoids is recommended initially [48].

Valvular calcification

Similar to valvulitis, calcification of the valves can result in both regurgitation and stenosis. Calcification can be present on any of the cardiac valves, but in the RA population is more commonly found on left-sided valves. In the general population, both cardiac valvular and arterial calcification are thought to be related to inflammation, although the exact mechanism remains unclear. A study using multi-detector computed tomography noted that patients with RA have a higher prevalence of both mitral and aortic valve calcification relative to their non-RA peers. Similar to the non-RA cohort, the presence of aortic and mitral valve calcification increases with age, although valve calcification is seen at younger ages in the RA population compared with the non-RA population. Age and duration of disease have been demonstrated as independent predictors of mitral valve calcification in RA patients. CRP has not been shown to be related to the presence of valvular calcification [49].

Rheumatoid nodules

Unlike fibrosis and calcification, rheumatoid nodules are more specific to systemic inflammatory diseases, particularly RA. Rheumatoid nodules in the heart are significantly less common than articular rheumatoid nodules but have been described on all four cardiac valves (Figure 2.5A and B). Rheumatoid nodules are most commonly found within and at the base of leaflets and valve rings, and less commonly on papillary muscles or endocardium. The presence of rheumatoid nodules on cardiac valves results in both stenosis and regurgitation (Figure 2.6). There is limited evidence that some cardiac rheumatoid nodules may improve with steroid therapy [50].

Non-infectious endocarditis

Although often associated with other rheumatologic conditions, non-infectious or autoimmune endocarditis is a particularly devastating complication of RA. It is a significant cause of valve damage and embolic phenomena. Autoimmune endocarditis is characterized by antibody-initiated damage and activation of the endothelium, followed by inflammatory cell infiltration with T cells and macrophages. The condition nonbacterial thrombotic endocarditis (NBTE) in which vegetations composed of platelet-fibrin thrombi develop on the valve, has also been described in RA. A specific subset of NBTE is Libman-Sacks endocarditis, which is commonly associated with systemic lupus erythematosus and antiphospholipid syndrome, but can also be present in RA. NBTE can result in valvular dysfunction or embolic disease requiring valve repair or replacement, although it can also be asymptomatic and identified only at autopsy [51].

Relationship to disease activity

Patients may have cardiac involvement with their RA but without cardiac symptoms or evidence of other extra-articular manifestations of RA. One of the challenges in characterizing VHD in RA patients is that disease

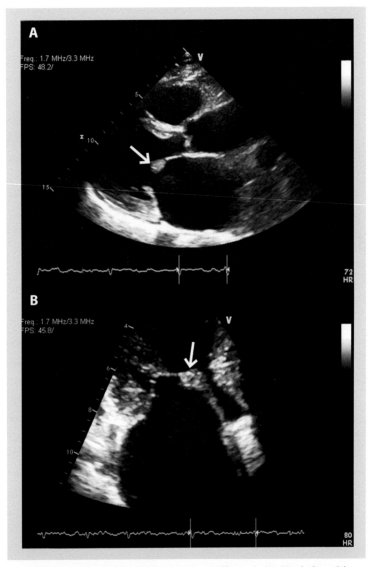

Figure 2.5 (A) Transthoracic echocardiogram, parasternal long axis view. Mitral valve nodule (arrow) on the tip of the anterior mitral valve leaflet in a patient with rheumatoid arthritis. **(B) Apical long axis view in the same patient, zoomed up on the mitral valve.** Anterior mitral valve leaflet with evidence of a nodule (arrow).

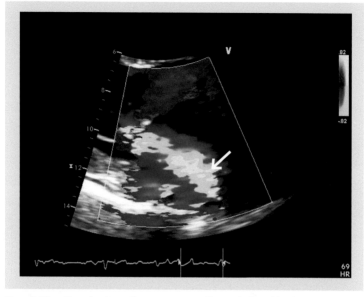

Figure 2.6 Transthoracic echocardiogram, parasternal long axis view with colour Doppler across the mitral valve showing mitral regurgitation (arrow) in the same patient as Figure 2.5.

activity is variable over time, but valvular disease is progressive. Thus, cross-sectional studies designed to evaluate the relationship between disease severity and the presence of VHD are forced to evaluate disease activity based on current markers of disease activity as opposed to lifetime cumulative disease activity. Several studies have failed to consistently identify any markers of disease activity or demographic characteristics that correspond to VHD [52].

Valve surgery in rheumatoid arthritis

Although much of the valvular heart disease in RA patients is asymptomatic, some patients will be hemodynamically compromised secondary to their valve disease and require surgery. Surgical treatment of VHD in RA patients requires a team approach, with involvement of the patient's rheumatologist, cardiologist, and cardio-thoracic surgeon. When a valve requires surgical replacement the health care team must select between a bioprosthetic or a mechanical valve. Mechanical valves provide a durable, long-lasting prosthesis. However, they promote valvular thrombotic vegetations and therefore require lifelong anticoagulation. This can be particularly problematic in patients with RA as these patients may require several joint surgeries, and they are prone to secondary antiphospholipid syndrome, with the increased risk for both thrombotic and bleeding complications. Alternatively, bioprosthetic valves have the benefit of not requiring long-term anticoagulation, which is favorable in patients who will need future orthopedic surgeries secondary to erosive RA. However, bioprosthetic valves have a limited life span, which may be even shorter in RA patients due to systemic inflammation. Data on cardiac surgery in antiphospholipid syndrome are limited to small case series, with conflicting results on whether it is better to replace with a bioprosthetic or a mechanical heart valve [53]. Many patients with RA have known antiphospholipid antibodies without overt antiphospholipid syndrome. The role of the presence of these antibodies in selecting a cardiac valve is unclear.

In addition to selecting a cardiac valve, perioperative management should include a multidisciplinary approach to managing both RA and cardiac symptoms. A database study that reviewed mitral valve procedure outcomes in RA patients found that RA patients have a similar length of stay and mortality relative to their non-RA peers undergoing similar procedures [54]. The presence of RA is not a contraindication to undergoing valve surgery.

References

1   Gordon DA, Stein JL, Broder I. The extra-articular features of rheumatoid arthritis. A systematic analysis of 127 cases. *Am J Med*. 1973;54:445-452.
2   Corrao S, Messina S, Pistone G, Calvo L, Scaglione R, Licata G. Heart involvement in rheumatoid arthritis: Systematic review and meta-analysis. *Int J Cardiol*. 2013;167:2031-2038.
3   Hara KS, Ballard DJ, Ilstrup DM, Connolly DC, Vollertsen RS. Rheumatoid pericarditis: clinical features and survival. *Medicine (Baltimore)*. 1990;69920:81-91.
4   Voskuyl AE. The heart and cardiovascular manifestations in rheumatoid arthritis. *Rheumatology (Oxford)*. 2006;45:iv4-iv7.
5   Jurik AG, Graudal H. Pericarditis in rheumatoid arthritis. A clinical and radiological study. *Rheumatol Int*. 1986;6:37-42.
6   Nomeir AM, Turner RA, Watts LE. Cardiac involvement in rheumatoid arthritis. Followup study. *Arthritis Rheum*. 1979;22:561-564.
7   Barcin C, Yalcinkaya E, Kabul HK. Cholesterol pericarditis associated with rheumatoid arthritis: a rare cause of pericardial effusion. *Int J Cardiol*. 2013;166:e56-e58.
8   Mitchell DM, Spitz PW, Young DY, Bloch DA, McShane DJ, Fries JF. Survival, prognosis, and causes of death in rheumatoid arthritis. *Arthritis Rheum*. 1986;29:706-714.

9 Edwards MH, Leak AM. Pericardial effusions on anti-tnf therapy for rheumatoid arthritis--a drug side effect or uncontrolled systemic disease? *Rheumatology (Oxford)*. 2009;48:316-317.

10 Harney S, O'Shea FD, FitzGerald O. Peptostreptococcal pericarditis complicating anti-tumour necrosis factor alpha treatment in rheumatoid arthritis. *Ann Rheum Dis*. 2002;61:653-654.

11 Lutman C, Finocchiaro G, Abate E, Milo M, Morassi P, Sinagra G. Purulent pericarditis in rheumatoid arthritis treated with rituximab and methotrexate. *J Cardiovasc Med (Hagerstown)*. 2014;15912):880-882.

12 Imazio M, Gaita F, LeWinter M. Evaluation and treatment of pericarditis. A systematic review. *JAMA*. 2015;314:1498-1506.

13 Jain S, Thongprayoon C, Espinosa RE, et al. Effectiveness and safety of anakinra for management of refractory pericarditis. *Am J Cardiol*. 2015;116:1277-1279.

14 Lebowitz WB. The heart in rheumatoid arthritis (rheumatoid disease). A clinical and pathological study of sixty-two cases. *Ann Intern Med*. 1963;58:102-123.

15 Bonfiglio T, Atwater EC. Heart disease in patients with seropositive rheumatoid arthritis; a controlled autopsy study and review. *Arch Intern Med*. 1969;124:714-719.

16 Abbas A, Byrd BF, 3rd. Right-sided heart failure due to right ventricular cavity obliteration by rheumatoid nodules. *Am J Cardiol*. 2000;86:711-712.

17 Mavrogeni S, Sfikakis PP, Karabela G, et al. Cardiovascular magnetic resonance imaging in asymptomatic patients with connective tissue disease and recent onset left bundle branch block. *Int J Cardiol*. 2014;171:82-87.

18 Guedes C, Bianchi-Fior P, Cormier B, Barthelemy B, Rat AC, Boissier MC. Cardiac manifestations of rheumatoid arthritis: A case-control transesophageal echocardiography study in 30 patients. *Arthritis Rheum*. 2001;45:129-135.

19 Steel KE, Kwong RY. Application of cardiac magnetic resonance imaging in cardiomyopathy. *Curr Heart Fail Rep*. 2008;5:128-135.

20 Puntmann VO, Taylor PC, Barr A, Schnackenburg B, Jahnke C, Paetsch I. Towards understanding the phenotypes of myocardial involvement in the presence of self-limiting and sustained systemic inflammation: a magnetic resonance imaging study. *Rheumatology (Oxford)*. 2010;49:528-535.

21 Slack JD, Waller B. Acute congestive heart failure due to the arteritis of rheumatoid arthritis: early diagnosis by endomyocardial biopsy: A case report. *Angiology*. 1986;37:477-482.

22 Seferovic PM, Ristic AD, Maksimovic R, et al. Cardiac arrhythmias and conduction disturbances in autoimmune rheumatic diseases. *Rheumatology (Oxford)*. 2006;45:iv39-iv42.

23 Singh JA, Furst DE, Bharat A, et al. 2012 Update of the 2008 American College of Rheumatology recommendations for the use of disease-modifying antirheumatic drugs and biologic agents in the treatment of rheumatoid arthritis. *Arthritis Care Res (Hoboken)*. 2012;64:625-639.

24 Joyce E, Fabre A, Mahon N. Hydroxychloroquine cardiotoxicity presenting as a rapidly evolving biventricular cardiomyopathy: Key diagnostic features and literature review. *Eur Heart J Acute Cardiovasc Care*. 2013;2:77-83.

25 Yogasundaram H, Putko BN, Tien J, et al. Hydroxychloroquine-induced cardiomyopathy: Case report, pathophysiology, diagnosis, and treatment. *Can J Cardiol*. 2014;30:1706-1715.

26 Rahman JE, Helou EF, Gelzer-Bell R, et al. Noninvasive diagnosis of biopsy-proven cardiac amyloidosis. *J Am Coll Cardiol*. 2004;43:410-415.

27 Selvanayagam JB, Hawkins PN, Paul B, Myerson SG, Neubauer S. Evaluation and management of the cardiac amyloidosis. *J Am Coll Cardiol*. 2007;50:2101-2110.

28 Perugini E, Rapezzi C, Piva T, et al. Non-invasive evaluation of the myocardial substrate of cardiac amyloidosis by gadolinium cardiac magnetic resonance. *Heart*. 2006;92:343-349.

29 Hattori Y, Ubara Y, Sumida K, et al. Tocilizumab improves cardiac disease in a hemodialysis patient with aa amyloidosis secondary to rheumatoid arthritis. *Amyloid*. 2012;19:37-40.

30 Wada Y, Kobayashi D, Murakami S, et al. Cardiac AA amyloidosis in a patient with rheumatoid arthritis and systemic sclerosis: the therapeutic potential of biological reagents. *Scand J Rheumatol*. 2011;40:402-404.

31 Mason JC, Libby P. Cardiovascular disease in patients with chronic inflammation: mechanisms underlying premature cardiovascular events in rheumatologic conditions. *Eur Heart J.* 2015;36:482-489c.

32 Hollan I, Meroni PL, Ahearn JM, et al. Cardiovascular disease in autoimmune rheumatic diseases. *Autoimmun Rev.* 2013;12:1004-1015.

33 Prasad M, Hermann J, Gabriel SE, et al. Cardiorheumatology: Cardiac involvement in systemic rheumatic disease. *Nat Rev Cardiol.* 2015;12:168-176.

34 Lazzerini PE, Capecchi PL, Acampa M, Galeazzi M, Laghi-Pasini F. Arrhythmic risk in rheumatoid arthritis: the driving role of systemic inflammation. *Autoimmun Rev.* 2014;13:936-944.

35 Guo Y, Lip GY, Apostolakis S. Inflammation in atrial fibrillation. *J Am Coll Cardiol.* 2012;60: 2263-2270.

36 Schnabel RB, Larson MG, Yamamoto JF, et al. Relation of multiple inflammatory biomarkers to incident atrial fibrillation. *Am J Cardiol.* 2009;104:92-96.

37 Yavuzkir M, Ozturk A, Dagli N, et al. Effect of ongoing inflammation in rheumatoid arthritis on p-wave dispersion. *J Int Med Res.* 2007;35:796-802.

38 Turgut O, Tandogan I, Yilmaz MB, Yalta K, Aydin O. Association of p wave duration and dispersion with the risk for atrial fibrillation: practical considerations in the setting of coronary artery disease. *Int J Cardiol.* 2010;144:322-324.

39 Lindhardsen J, Ahlehoff O, Gislason GH, et al. Risk of atrial fibrillation and stroke in rheumatoid arthritis: Danish nationwide cohort study. *BMJ.* 2012;344:e1257.

40 Kim SC, Liu J, Solomon DH. The risk of atrial fibrillation in patients with rheumatoid arthritis. *Ann Rheum Dis.* 2014;73:1091-1095.

41 Bacani AK, Crowson CS, Roger VL, Gabriel SE, Matteson EL. Increased incidence of atrial fibrillation in patients with rheumatoid arthritis. *BioMed Res Internat.* 2015;2015:809514.

42 Jurik AG, Moller P. Atrioventricular conduction time in rheumatoid arthritis. *Rheumatol Int.* 1985;5:205-207.

43 Maradit-Kremers H, Crowson CS, Nicola PJ, et al. Increased unrecognized coronary heart disease and sudden deaths in rheumatoid arthritis: A population-based cohort study. *Arthritis Rheum.* 2005;52:402-411.

44 Chauhan K, Ackerman MJ, Crowson CS, Matteson EL, Gabriel SE. Population-based study of QT interval prolongation in patients with rheumatoid arthritis. *Clin Exp Rheumatol.* 2015;33:84-89.

45 Panoulas VF, Toms TE, Douglas KM, et al. Prolonged QTc interval predicts all-cause mortality in patients with rheumatoid arthritis: An association driven by high inflammatory burden. *Rheumatology (Oxford).* 2014;53:131-137.

46 Lazzerini PE, Acampa M, Capecchi PL, et al. Association between high sensitivity c-reactive protein, heart rate variability and corrected QT interval in patients with chronic inflammatory arthritis. *Eur J Intern Med.* 2013;24:368-374.

47 Sen D, González-Mayda M, Brasington RD Jr. Cardiovascular disease in rheumatoid arthritis. *Rheum Dis Clin North Am.* 2014;40:27-49.

48 Kaneko S, Yamashita H, Sugimori Y, et al. Rheumatoid arthritis-associated aortitis: a case report and literature review. *Springerplus.* 2014;3:509

49 Yiu KH, Wang S, Mok MY, et al. Relationship between cardiac valvular and arterial calcification in patients with rheumatoid arthritis and systemic lupus erythematosus. *J Rheumatol.* 2011;38:621-627.

50 Maksimowicz-McKinnon K, Mandell BF. Understanding valvular heart disease in patients with systemic autoimmune diseases. *Cleve Clin J Med.* 2004;71:881-885.

51 Eiken PW, Edwards WD, Tazelaar HD, McBane RD, Zehr KJ. Surgical pathology of nonbacterial thrombotic endocarditis in 30 patients, 1985-2000. *Mayo Clin Proc.* 2001;76:1204-1212.

52 Beckhauser AP, Vallin L, Burkievcz CJ, Perreto S, Silva MB, Skare TL. Valvular involvement in patients with rheumatoid arthritis. *Acta Reumatol Port.* 2009;34:52-56.

53 Erdozain JG, Ruiz-Irastorza G, Segura MI, et al. Cardiac valve replacement in patients with antiphospholipid syndrome. *Arthritis Care Res(Hoboken).* 2012;64:1256-1260.

54 Vassileva CM, Kwedar K, Boley T, Markwell S, Hazelrigg S. Mitral valve procedure selection and outcomes in patients with rheumatoid arthritis. J Heart Valve Dis. 2013;22:14-19

Chapter 3

Risk factors for cardiovascular disease in rheumatoid arthritis

Theodoros Dimitroulas and George Kitas

The reasons for the increased cardiovascular disease (CVD) risk in rheumatoid arthritis (RA) have not been determined. The presence of traditional CVD risk factors such as abnormal lipid metabolism, hypertension, obesity, and smoking cannot fully explain the higher incidence of CVD events in this population [1]. Novel risk factors such as systemic inflammation and autoimmune activation have been identified as important players in the development of premature atherosclerosis. In fact, epidemiological evidence suggests that inflammation correlates with cardiovascular events and confers a statistically significant increased risk for CVD deaths in patients with RA [2]. Clinical and serological features of severe, uncontrolled RA such as high inflammatory markers, rheumatoid factor positivity, large joint swelling, and extra-articular involvement are highly significant predictors of cardiovascular outcome and mortality [3]. Such observations underline the complex interrelations between traditional, novel, and disease-related risk factors all of which contribute to heightened CVD risk in patients with RA .

In this chapter we focus on hypertension, lipid profile, and insulin resistance/diabetes as contributors to the increased CVD risk in RA and discuss the impact of systemic inflammation and disease activity on CVD complications in this population.

© Springer International Publishing Switzerland 2017
A.G. Semb (ed.), *Handbook of Cardiovascular Disease Management in Rheumatoid Arthritis*, DOI 10.1007/978-3-319-26782-1_3

Traditional cardiovascular risk factors in patients with rheumatoid arthritis

Conventional CVD risk factors are strong predictors of CVD events and outcomes in the general population, but their impact on CVD morbidity and mortality in RA remains only partly understood. RA patients tend to have a different profile of risk factors compared with the general population, which is associated with higher frequency of smoking, unfavorable total cholesterol/HDL ratio, hypertension, and insulin resistance [4]. However, studies examining the distribution of classic CVD risk factors amongst RA and non-RA individuals provide somewhat contradictory results. Reports from different groups [5,6] have demonstrated that the incidence of many of the traditional CVD risk factors is similar between RA and non-RA subjects, while others have found increased prevalence of – unrecognized and/or undertreated - hypertension, high lipid levels, and diabetes mellitus within RA populations [7–9]. Even if classic CVD risk factors are equally or only slightly more prevalent in RA, there are notable differences in the way they influence CVD outcomes with some of the risk factors displaying paradoxical effects and associations [10]. For example low body mass index (BMI) is associated with increased CVD risk among RA patients but not in non-RA individuals, because low BMI in RA may reflect body composition changes due to increased disease activity. It has been suggested that classical CVD risk factors operate differently in RA patients and the general population as systemic inflammation modulates the adverse effects of such risk factors on vasculature. This concurs with published data suggesting that the relative impact of several traditional risk factors on CVD was less in RA subjects compared with those who do not have RA [11]. Other studies have shown that the importance of the traditional risk factors regarding risk of CVD morbidity in patients with RA has been shown to be comparable to what is reported for the general population. A meta-analysis revealed that traditional risk factors independently increase the risk of CVD morbidity in RA; hypertension (relative risk [RR] 2.24, 95% confidence interval [CI] 1.42, 3.06), hypercholesterolemia (RR 1.73, 95% CI 1.03, 2.44), diabetes mellitus (RR 1.94, 95% CI 1.58, 2.30), smoking (RR1.50, 95% CI 1.15, 1.84), and obesity (RR 1.16, 95% CI 1.03, 1.29)[12]. In addition, recent findings indicate that classic CVD risk factors are better predictors of abnormal vascular function and morphology than current and/or cumulative inflammatory load in RA [13,14], underscoring their important role in the initiation of vascular injury and highlighting the need for CVD prevention and management strategies in this population.

Hypertension

Hypertension is an important modifiable risk factor for the development of CVD in the general population [15] and the risk of CVD morbidity can be reduced with a modest reduction in blood pressure (3–5 mmHg). There are contradictory reports regarding whether hypertension is more common in RA compared with the general population (Table 3.1) [16–19]. However in a recent study Chung et al [7] found that undiagnosed hypertension was more common in RA patients compared with controls. According to a systematic review the prevalence of hypertension in RA patients lies between 52% and 73%; the wide range of reported incidence can be attributed to differences in study populations assessed, varied sample sizes, and the definition of hypertension used [20]. High blood pressure appears to be a major player in increasing CVD risk in RA as it associates with subclinical atherosclerosis [21] and has been characterized as one of the most important independent predictors of CVD events

Study [reference]	Number of patients	Study type	Hypertension prevalence (%)	Undiagnosed (%)
Chung et al [7]	197 RA / 274 controls	Cross-sectional	113 (57 %) RA vs 115 (42%) controls	NC
Panoulas et al [16]	400 RA	Cross-sectional	282 (71%)	39%
Maradit-Kremers et al [17]	603 RA/ 603 controls	Cross-sectional	314 (51%) RA vs 241 (40%) controls	NC
Dougados et al [18]	3920 RA	Cross-sectional	1568 (40%)	NC
Dessein et al [19]	79 RA	Cross-sectional	39 (50%)	NC
Protogerou et al [24]	214 RA	Cross-sectional	116 (54%)	10%

Table 3.1 Prevalence of hypertension in rheumatoid arthritis according to different studies.
NC, not characterized, RA, rheumatoid arthritis; vs, versus.

with relative risk ranging from between 1.49 to 4.3 [22,23]. Despite the growing appreciation regarding the important role of hypertension in the increased CVD risk amongst patients with RA, high blood pressure still remains underdiagnosed and poorly controlled within this population [16, 24]. Thus, it is not surprising that unrecognized and untreated hypertension is associated with more frequent and severe target organ damage in RA [25].

A multitude of interrelated factors may be contributing to the high prevalence of hypertension in RA patients, including physical inactivity [26]. RA itself can also be a risk factor for the development of hypertension through various mechanisms (Figure 3.1). Systemic inflammation affects nitric oxide production leading to endothelial dysfunction, vasoconstriction, and vascular damage promoting atherosclerosis and hypertension [27]. In addition, chronic inflammation results in arterial stiffness as RA patients demonstrate reduced small- and large-artery elasticity and greater systemic vascular resistance compared with age- and

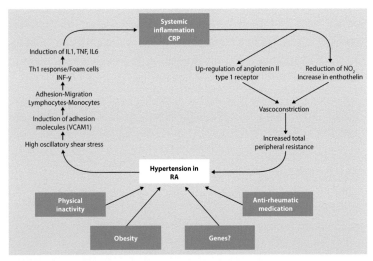

Figure 3.1 The interplay between rheumatoid arthritis-related factors and derangement of vascular physiology leading to hypertension. Vascular and systemic inflammation affect each other resulting in endothelial dysfunction, vasoconstriction, and high blood pressure. A sedentary life style also contributes to hypertension as well as several immunosuppressive regimens. CRP, C-reactive protein; IL-1/6, interleukin1/6; NO, nitric oxide; Th, T-helper lymphocytes; VCAM, vascular cell adhesion molecule. Reproduced with permission from © Oxford University Press, 2008. All Rights Reserved. Panoulas et al [20].

sex-matched controls [28], which may subsequently lead to higher values of central blood pressure. In the general population, it has been shown to be an association between chronic-low grade inflammation – assessed by high sensitivity CRP–and hypertension [29], which has not been confirmed in RA [16]. This unresolved issue remains to be addressed in prospective studies.

Disease modifying anti-rheumatic medications (DMARDs) and other drugs used for the management of RA can also induce high blood pressure. Non-steroidal anti-inflammatory drugs (NSAIDs) leflunomide and cyclosporine have significant hypertensive effects and prescription of these medications, particularly in patients with hypertension, should be decided cautiously and preferably after ensuring the 24-hour average blood pressure is achieved by use of blood pressure surveillance systems. Corticosteroids may also contribute to the development of hypertension. However, it remains unknown whether the higher prevalence of hypertension documented in patients receiving a medium dose of prednisolone (≤7.5 mg/day) is attributable to the medication itself or can be explained on the basis of higher inflammatory burden observed in patients requiring regular treatment with steroids [16].

Lipids

The relationship between lipids and risk of CVD in RA patients is complex. In the general population, a nearly linear relationship between cholesterol and risk of CVD is well-established. Although, increased lipid levels have been shown to be common and affect between 55% and 65% of RA patients in one UK cohort [30], patients with RA generally have lower lipid levels compared with non-RA persons. It may be that the lipid/CVD risk curve is U-shaped, because low lipid levels in RA also confer high CVD risk; this has been termed the lipid paradox. Despite lower lipid levels in RA patients compared with non-RA subjects in the AMORIS study, RA patients had a higher risk of both myocardial infarction and ischemic stroke compared with non-RA subjects [31]. The increased risk of CVD at low lipid levels may be confounded by inflammation, considering a reported significant interaction between low density lipoprotein cholesterol (LDL-c) and erythrocyte sedimentation rate (ESR) [32]. Acute or chronic high-grade inflammation results in the suppression of total cholesterol with a proportionately greater suppression of high-density lipoprotein cholesterol (HDL-c), which yields an increased and unfavorable total cholesterol:HDL-c ratio. This may better reflect the actual risk of CVD in RA patients than use of the individual lipid parameters [33].

Retrospective studies have reported abnormal lipoprotein patterns even 10 years prior to the onset of RA [34] suggesting that lower lipid levels may render people more susceptible to development of RA. It remains unknown whether these changes in lipids are associated with the pro-inflammatory state present many years before the clinical manifestations of RA or with the genetic background. Toms et al [35] reported an association between RA susceptibility genes and low lipid levels in RA patients. These findings have later been confirmed by Liao and colleagues reporting that RA risk alleles were also found to be linked to lower LDL-c [36].

In the general population HDL-c takes part in reverse cholesterol transport of LDL-c from the periphery (atherosclerotic plaque) to the liver. HDL-c also entails anti-inflammatory and other anti-atherosclerotic properties. It has been shown that increasing levels of HDL-c have a cardioprotective effect. Although, data indicate that the cardioprotective effect of HDL-c is also U-shaped because both high [37] and low [38] HDL-levels do not confer a benefit against CVD events. Furthermore, the functional properties of HDL-c have been shown to be influenced by inflammation and the interactions between systemic inflammation and abnormal lipid metabolism are complex. Inflammatory mediators and cytokines, such as tumor necrosis factor-alpha (TNF-α) and interleukin-6 (IL-6), act in adipose tissue, liver, and skeletal muscle to promote changes in lipid metabolism (Figure 3.2). The level of HDL-c has been shown to be related to IL-6 [39] while other acute phase proteins such as serum amyloid A and phospholipase A2 have been reported to cause structural and functional changes of HDL-c, altering its anti-atherogenic functions [40]. Systemic inflammation may influence HDL-c properties and composition by various mechanisms, converting it to a more pro-oxidant molecule [41]. Antirheumatic medication such as biologic DMARDs (bDMARDs), dampening inflammation, may also restore the

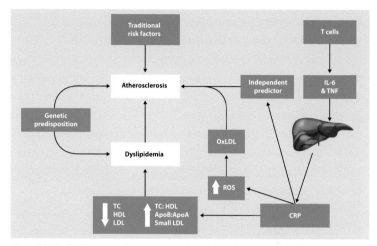

Figure 3.2 Mechanisms contributing to pro-atherosclerotic changes in lipids in rheumatoid arthritis. Systemic inflammation influences lipid metabolism in liver and adipose tissue leading to an unfavorable TC/HDL ratio. ApoB:ApoA, apolipoprotein B:apolipoprotein A; CRP, C-reactive protein; HDL, high-density lipoproteins; IL-6, interleukin 6; OxLDL, oxidized low-density lipoproteins; ROS, reactive oxygen species; TC, total cholesterol; TNF, tumour necrosis factor. Reproduced with permission from © Bentham Open, 2011. All Rights Reserved. Toms et al [43].

HDL functions [42]. Adding to this complexity, the fact that conventional and bDMARDs as well as lifestyle factors such as physical inactivity and obesity also affect lipid levels and function; it is clear that further research is required to investigate this interplay.

Insulin resistance and diabetes

RA shares numerous pathophysiological processes with the metabolic syndrome, such as high blood pressure, obesity, low HDL-c, and high triglyceride levels [44]. Insulin resistance is one of the main components of the metabolic syndrome and it is an important contributor to the CVD risk. The chronic low-grade inflammation present in the metabolic syndrome and the multiple pleiotropic effects of adipokines on the vasculature has been implicated in the pathogenesis of vascular injury in RA patients [45]. It is now well-recognized and accepted that the magnitude of CVD risk in RA is comparable to that of diabetes mellitus [46,47]. In patients with RA also having diabetes, the risk of CVD is nearly doubled compared with RA patients without diabetes [47].

The impact of rheumatoid arthritis disease activity and severity on cardiovascular comorbidity

Electrophysiological and structural function of the heart has been shown to be affected by disease activity (Table 3.2). Autonomic heart dysfunction and echocardiographic indices of left ventricular remodeling have been shown to correlate with disease severity in cross-sectional studies [48–50]. In addition, several lines of evidence suggest a link

Study	Patients/ subjects	Study type	Parameters assessed	Assessment tools	Associations
Midtbo et al [48]	129 RA/102 controls	Cross-sectional	LV relative wall thickness	Echo-cardiography	High disease activity (SDAI >3.3)/LV wall thickness
Lazzerini et al [49]	101 RA	Cross-sectional	HRV and QT interval	15-minute ambulatory 12-channel electrocardio-gram	CRP/HRV and QT intervals
Panoulas et al [50]	357 RA	Cross-sectional	QT corrected interval	Electro-cardiography	CRP/ QT corrected interval
Del Rincon et al [51]	204 RA	Cross-sectional	Carotid artery IMT	Carotid ultrasound	ESR/IMT
Gonzalez-Gay et al [52]	47 RA	Cross-sectional	Carotid artery IMT	Carotid ultrasound	CRP/IMT
Semb et al [53]	152 RA/89 controls	Cross-sectional	Vulnerability of carotid plaques	Carotid ultrasound Gray-scale median technique	Vulnerable carotid plaques/ high disease activity
Myasoedova et al [57]	525 RA/524 controls	Longitudinal	Cumulative burden of RA disease severity	RARBIS, CIRAS	Cumulative burden of RA disease severity/CVD events
Solomon et al [58]	24989 RA	Longitudinal	Time averaged disease activity	CDAI	↓ CDAI/ ↓ CVD risk

Table 3.2 Associations between disease activity and cardiovascular disease risk in rheumatoid arthritis. CDAI, clinical disease activity index; CIRAS, claims-based index of RA severity; CRP, C-reactive protein; CVD, cardiovascular events; ESR, Erythrocyte sedimentation rate; HRV, heart rate variability; IMT, intima-media thickness; LV, left ventricle; RA, rheumatoid arthritis; RARBIS, records-based index of severity; SDAI, simplified disease activity index.

between accelerated atherosclerosis and disease activity. For example, inflammatory markers such as ESR and CRP have been associated with morphological markers of subclinical atherosclerosis [51,52]. Carotid atherosclerotic plaque vulnerability has been shown to be associated with moderate/high disease activity in RA patients compared with patients in remission and non-RA subjects [53]. Subclinical disease activity and age >55 years of age were described as the sole predictors of coronary artery plaque vulnerability in RA patients [54], confirming previous reports underlying the higher probability of acute CVD events in patients with severe, uncontrolled disease. However, this evidence is mainly based on a single-point determination of RA activity measure, which obviously does not precisely reflect the magnitude of the inflammatory response over time. Patients with longer periods of severe disease are more likely to develop CVD complications possibly due to the effect of accumulated inflammatory burden on the vasculature [55,56].

In this regard, Myasoedova et al described the association of RA disease flare and higher cumulative burden of RA severity with CVD occurrence, using population-based longitudinal data [57]. Similar observations were made in a large cohort of almost 25,000 patients after a median follow-up period of 2.7 years, in whom lower disease activity was accompanied by a trend towards reduced risk of CVD events [58]. In contrast, disease duration does not appear to have the same effect on CVD risk [59] and such findings underscore the importance of tight, sustained control of systemic inflammation not only for the improvement of functional status but also for the reduction of CVD risk.

The role of inflammation in the development of cardiovascular disease manifestations of rheumatoid arthritis

The role of systemic inflammation as an additional contributor to the excess CVD risk in RA, is increasingly appreciated. Levels of CRP and ESR have been linked with heightened CVD morbidity in both the general population [60] and RA individulas even after adjusting for traditional CVD risk factors [61]. Inflammatory processes in the rheumatoid synovium and atherosclerotic plaques are remarkably similar, suggesting that the intensity of vascular inflammation is an important factor to the development of accelerated atherosclerosis in RA. Although the exact mechanism by which rheumatic inflammation and atherosclerosis influence each other remains to be determined, growing evidence supports the notion that pro-inflammatory cytokines such as TNF-alpha and IL-6 disrupt endothelial hemostasis leading to vascular dysfunction – an early step in atherogenesis [27]. The impaired vascular function and morphology in RA patients lacks a clear association with systemic inflammatory burden [62]. In addition, systemic inflammation contributes to abnormal fibrinolytic activity and enhances prothrombotic propensity in RA patients [63], playing a crucial role in thrombus formation. In conclusion, chronic high-grade systemic inflammation precipitates adverse effects of traditional CVD risk factors on the vascular wall, underlining the complexity of the links between RA-related factors and impairment of endothelial function (Figure 3.3) [64].

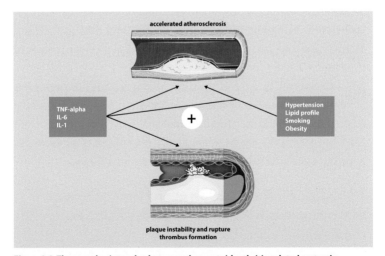

Figure 3.3 The complex interplay between rheumatoid arthritis-related systemic inflammation and traditional cardiovascular disease risk factors in rheumatoid arthritis. Systemic inflammation precipitates the adverse effects of traditional cardiovascular disease risk factors on vascular wall directly and/or indirectly. More importantly the magnitude of chronic inflammation may be a main contributor of plaque instability and hypercoagulable state resulting in plaque rupture and thrombosis/clot formation. IL-1, interleukin-1; IL-6, interleukin-6; TNF, tumor necrosis factor.

References

1   van den Oever IA, van Sijl AM, Nurmohamed MT. Management of cardiovascular risk in patients with rheumatoid arthritis: evidence and expert opinion. *Ther Adv Musculoskelet Dis.* 2013;5:166-181.

2   Solomon DH, Curhan GC, Rimm EB, Cannuscio CC, Karlson EW. Cardiovascular risk factors in women with and without rheumatoid arthritis. *Arthritis Rheum.* 2004;50:3444-3449.

3   Gabriel SE. Why do people with rheumatoid arthritis still die prematurely? *Ann Rheum Dis.* 2008;67:iii30-iii34.

4   Van Breukelen-van der Stoep DF, Klop B, van Zeben D, Hazes JM, Castro CabezasM. Cardiovascular risk in rheumatoid arthritis: how to lower the risk? *Atherosclerosis.* 2013;231:163-172.

5   Gonzalez A, Maradit-Kremers H, Crowson CS,et al. Do cardiovascular risk factors confer the same risk for cardiovascular outcomes in rheumatoid arthritis patients as in non-rheumatoid arthritis patients? *Ann Rheum Dis.* 2008;67:64-69.

6   Solomon DH, Curhan GC, Rimm EB, Cannuscio CC, Karlson EW. Cardiovascular risk factors in women with and without rheumatoid arthritis. *Arthritis Rheum.* 2004;50:3444-3449.

7   Chung CP, Giles JT, Petri M, Szklo M, Post W, Blumenthal RS, et al. Prevalence of traditional modifiable cardiovascular risk factors in patients with rheumatoid arthritis: comparison with control subjects from the multi-ethnic study of atherosclerosis. *Semin Arthritis Rheum.* 2012;41:535-544.

8   Erb N, Pace AV, Douglas KM, Banks MJ, Kitas GD. Risk assessment for coronary heart disease in rheumatoid arthritis and osteoarthritis. *Scand J Rheumatol.* 2004;33:293-299.

9   Boyer JF, Gourraud PA, Cantagrel A, Davignon JL, Constantin A. Traditional cardiovascular risk factors in rheumatoid arthritis: a meta-analysis. *Joint Bone Spine.* 2011;78:179-183.

10 Solomon DH, Kremer J, Curtis JR, Hochberg MC, Reed G, Tsao P, et al. Explaining the cardiovascular risk associated with rheumatoid arthritis: traditional risk factors versus markers of rheumatoid arthritis severity. *Ann Rheum Dis.* 2010;69:1920-1925.

11 Gabriel SE. Heart disease and rheumatoid arthritis: understanding the risks. *Ann Rheum Dis.* 2010;69:i61-i64.

12 Baghdadi LR, Woodman RJ, Shanahan EM, Mangoni AA. The impact of traditional cardiovascular risk factors on cardiovascular outcomes in patients with rheumatoid arthritis: a systematic review and meta-analysis. *PLoS One.* 2015;10:e0117952.

13 Sandoo A, Kitas GD, Carroll D, Veldhuijzen van Zanten JJ. The role of inflammation and cardiovascular disease risk on microvascular and macrovascularendothelial function in patients with rheumatoid arthritis: a cross-sectional and longitudinal study. *Arthritis Res Ther.* 2012;14:R117.

14 Sandoo A, Chanchlani N, Hodson J, Smith JP, Douglas KM, Kitas GD. Classical cardiovascular disease risk factors associate with vascular function and morphology in rheumatoid arthritis: a six-year prospective study. *Arthritis Res Ther.* 2013;15:R203.

15 Yusuf S, Hawken S, Ounpuu S, et al. Effect of potentially modifiable risk factors associated with myocardial infarction in 52 countries (the INTERHEART study): case-control study. *Lancet.* 2004;364:937-952.

16 Panoulas VF, Douglas KM, Milionis HJ, et al. Prevalence and associations of hypertension and its control in patients with rheumatoid arthritis. *Rheumatology (Oxford).* 2007;46:1477-1482

17 Maradit-Kremers H, Nicola PJ, Crowson CS, Ballman KV, Gabriel SE. Cardiovascular death in rheumatoid arthritis: a population-based study. *Arthritis Rheum.* 2005;52:722-732.

18 Dougados M, Soubrier M, Antunez A, et al. Prevalence of comorbidities in rheumatoid arthritis and evaluation of their monitoring: results of an international, cross-sectional study (COMORA). *Ann Rheum Dis.* 2014;73:62-68.

19 Dessein PH, Stanwix AE, Joffe BI. Cardiovascular risk in rheumatoid arthritis versus osteoarthritis: acute phase response related decreased insulin sensitivity and high-density lipoprotein cholesterol as well as clustering of metabolic syndrome features in rheumatoid arthritis. *Arthritis Res.* 2002;4:R5.

20 Panoulas VF, Metsios GS, Pace AV, et al. Hypertension in rheumatoid arthritis. *Rheumatology (Oxford)*. 2008;47:1286-1298.

21 Gerli R, Sherer Y, Vaudo G, et al. Early atherosclerosis in rheumatoid arthritis: effects of smoking on thickness of the carotid artery intima media. *Ann N Y Acad Sci*. 2005;1051:281-290.

22 Assous N, Touzé E, Meune C, Kahan A, Allanore Y. Cardiovascular disease in rheumatoid arthritis: single-center hospital-based cohort study in France. *Joint Bone Spine*. 2007;74:66-72.

23 Wållberg-Jonsson S, Johansson H, Ohman ML, Rantapää-Dahlqvist S. Extent of inflammation predicts cardiovascular disease and overall mortality in seropositive rheumatoid arthritis. A retrospective cohort study from disease onset. *J Rheumatol*. 1999;26:2562-2571.

24 Protogerou AD, Panagiotakos DB, Zampeli E, et al. Arterial hypertension assessed "out-of-office" in a contemporary cohort of rheumatoid arthritis patients free of cardiovascular disease is characterized by high prevalence, low awareness, poor control and increased vascular damage-associated "white coat" phenomenon. *Arthritis Res Ther*. 2013;15:R142.

25 Panoulas VF, Toms TE, Metsios GS, et al. Target organ damage in patients with rheumatoid arthritis: the role of blood pressure and heart rate. *Atherosclerosis*. 2010;209:255-260.

26 Paffenbarger RS Jr, Lee IM. Intensity of physical activity related to incidence of hypertension and all-cause mortality: an epidemiological view. *Blood Press Monit*. 1997;2:115-123.

27 Mason JC, Libby P. Cardiovascular disease in patients with chronic inflammation: mechanisms underlying premature cardiovascular events in rheumatologic conditions. *Eur Heart J*. 2015;36:482-489c.

28 Wong M, Toh L, Wilson A, et al. Reduced arterial elasticity in rheumatoid arthritis and the relationship to vascular disease risk factors and inflammation. *Arthritis Rheum*. 2003;48:81-89.

29 Rohde LE, Hennekens CH, Ridker PM. Survey of C-reactive protein and cardiovascular risk factors in apparently healthy men. *Am J Cardiol*. 1999;84:1018-1022.

30 Toms TE, Symmons DP, Kitas GD. Dyslipidaemia in rheumatoid arthritis: the role of inflammation, drugs, lifestyle and genetic factors. *Curr Vasc Pharmacol*. 2010;8:301-326.

31 Semb AG, Kvien TK, Aastveit AH, et al. Lipids, myocardial infarction and ischaemic stroke in patients with rheumatoid arthritis in the Apolipoprotein-related Mortality RISk (AMORIS) Study. *Ann Rheum Dis*. 2010;69:1996-2001.

32 Myasoedova E, Crowson CS, Kremers HM, et al. Lipid paradox in rheumatoid arthritis: the impact of serum lipid measures and systemic inflammation on the risk of cardiovascular disease. *Ann Rheum Dis*. 2011;70:482-487.

33 Peters MJ, Voskuyl AE, Sattar N, Dijkmans BA, Smulders YM, Nurmohamed MT. The interplay between inflammation, lipids and cardiovascular risk in rheumatoid arthritis: why ratios may be better. *Int J Clin Pract*. 2010;64:1440-1443.

34 van Halm VP, Nielen MM, Nurmohamed MT, et al. Lipids and inflammation: serial measurements of the lipid profile of blood donors who later developed rheumatoid arthritis. *Ann Rheum Dis*. 2007;66:184-188.

35 Toms TE, Panoulas VF, Smith JP, et al. Rheumatoid arthritis susceptibility genes associate with lipid levels in patients with rheumatoid arthritis. *Ann Rheum Dis*. 2011;70:1025-1032.

36 Liao KP, Diogo D, Cui J, et al. Association between low density lipoprotein and rheumatoid arthritis genetic factors with low density lipoprotein levels in rheumatoid arthritis and non-rheumatoid arthritis controls. *Ann Rheum Dis*. 2014;73:1170-1175.

37 Ko DT, Alter DA, Guo H, et al. Relationship between high-density lipoprotein cholesterol and cardiovascular and non-cardiovascular mortality: a population-based study of more than 630,000 individuals without prior cardiovascular conditions in Ontario, Canada. American Heart Association Scientific Sessions 2015. http://www.abstractsonline.com/pp8/#!/3795/presentation/46013. Accessed February 4, 2016.

38 Kannel WB. High-density lipoproteins: epidemiologic profile and risks of coronary artery disease. *Am J Cardiol*. 1983;52:9B-12B.

39 Gomaraschi M, Basilico N, Sisto F, Taramelli D, Eligini S, Colli S, et al. High-density lipoproteins attenuate interleukin-6 production in endothelial cells exposed to pro-inflammatory stimuli. *Biochim Biophys Acta*. 2005;1736:136-143.

40 Watanabe J, Charles-Schoeman C, Miao Y, et al. Proteomic profiling following immune affinity capture of high-density lipoprotein: association of acute-phase proteins and complement factors with proinflammatory high-density lipoprotein in rheumatoid arthritis. *Arthritis Rheum*. 2012;64:1828-1837.

41 Charles-Schoeman C, Lee YY, Grijalva V, et al. Cholesterol efflux by high density lipoproteins is impaired in patients with active rheumatoid arthritis. *Ann Rheum Dis*. 2012;71:1157–1162.

42 Popa C, van Tits LJ, Barrera P, et al. Anti-inflammatory therapy with tumour necrosis factor alpha inhibitors improves high-density lipoprotein cholesterol antioxidative capacity in rheumatoid arthritis patients. *Ann Rheum Dis*. 2009;68:868-872.

43 Toms TE, Panoulas VF, Kitas GD. Dyslipidaemia in rheumatological autoimmune diseases. *Open Cardiovasc Med J*. 2011;5:64-75

44 Bilecik NA, Tuna S, Samancı N, Balcı N, Akbaş H. Prevalence of metabolic syndrome in women with rheumatoid arthritis and effective factors. *Int J Clin Exp Med*. 2014;7:2258-2265.

45 Ferraccioli G, Gremese E. Adiposity, joint and systemic inflammation: the additional risk of having a metabolic syndrome in rheumatoid arthritis. *Swiss Med Wkly*. 2011;141:w13211.

46 Stamatelopoulos KS, Kitas GD, Papamichael CM, et al. Atherosclerosis in rheumatoid arthritis versus diabetes: a comparative study. *Arterioscler Thromb Vasc Biol*. 2009;29:1702-1708.

47 Lindhardsen J, Ahlehoff O, Gislason GH, Madsen OR, Olesen JB, Torp-Pedersen C, Hansen PR. The risk of myocardial infarction in rheumatoid arthritis and diabetes mellitus: a Danish nationwide cohort study. *Ann Rheum Dis*. 2011;70:929-934.

48 Midtbo H, Gerdts E, Kvien TK, et al. Disease activity and left ventricular structure in patients with rheumatoid arthritis. *Rheumatology (Oxford)*. 2015;54:511-519.

49 Lazzerini PE, Acampa M, Capecchi PL, et al. Association between high sensitivity C-reactive protein, heart rate variability and corrected QT interval in patients with chronic inflammatory arthritis. *Eur J Intern Med*. 2013;24:368-374.

50 Panoulas VF, Toms TE, Douglas KM, Sandoo A, Metsios GS, Stavropoulos-Kalinoglou A, Kitas GD. Prolonged QTc interval predicts all-cause mortality in patients with rheumatoid arthritis: an association driven by high inflammatory burden. *Rheumatology (Oxford)*. 2014;53:131-137.

51 Del Rincón I, Williams K, Stern MP, Freeman GL, O'Leary DH, Escalante A. Association between carotid atherosclerosis and markers of inflammation in rheumatoid arthritis patients and healthy subjects. *Arthritis Rheum*. 2003;48:1833-1840.

52 Gonzalez-Gay MA, Gonzalez-Juanatey C, Piñeiro A, Garcia-Porrua C, Testa A, Llorca J. High-grade C-reactive protein elevation correlates with accelerated atherogenesis in patients with rheumatoid arthritis. *J Rheumatol*. 2005;32:1219-1223.

53 Semb AG, Rollefstad S, Provan SA, et al. Carotid plaque characteristics and disease activity in rheumatoid arthritis. *J Rheumatol*. 2013;40:359-368.

54 Karpouzas GA, Malpeso J, Choi TY, Li D, Munoz S, Budoff MJ. Prevalence, extent and composition of coronary plaque in patients with rheumatoid arthritis without symptoms or prior diagnosis of coronary artery disease. *Ann Rheum Dis*. 2014;73:1797-1804.

55 Sandoo A, Kitas GD. Current perspectives on the assessment of vascular function and morphology in rheumatoid arthritis. *Int J Clin Rheumatol*. 2013;8:1-3.

56 Sandoo A, Dimitroulas T, Hodson J, Smith JP, Douglas KM, Kitas GD. Cumulative inflammation associates with asymmetric dimethylarginine in rheumatoid arthritis: a 6 year follow-up study. *Rheumatology (Oxford)*. 2015;54:1145-1152.

57 Myasoedova E, Chandran A, Ilhan B, et al. The role of rheumatoid arthritis (RA) flare and cumulative burden of RA severity in the risk of cardiovascular disease. *Ann Rheum Dis*. 2015;pii: annrheumdis-2014-206411.

58 Solomon DH, Reed GW, Kremer JM, et al. Disease activity in rheumatoid arthritis and the risk of cardiovascular events. *Arthritis Rheumatol*. 2015;67:1449-1455.

59 Arts EE, Fransen J, den Broeder AA, Popa CD, van Riel PL. The effect of disease duration and disease activity on the risk of cardiovascular disease in rheumatoid arthritis patients. *Ann Rheum Dis*. 2015;74:998-1003.

60 Emerging Risk Factors Collaboration, Kaptoge S, Di Angelantonio E, et al. C-reactive protein concentration and risk of coronary heart disease, stroke, and mortality: an individual participant meta-analysis. *Lancet*. 2010;375:132-140.

61 Myasoedova E, Crowson CS, Green AB, Matteson EL, Gabriel SE. Longterm blood pressure variability in patients with rheumatoid arthritis and its effect on cardiovascular events and all-cause mortality in RA: a population-based comparative cohort study. *J Rheumatol*. 2014;41:1638-1644.

62 Sandoo A, Veldhuijzen van Zanten JJ, Metsios GS, Carroll D, Kitas GD. Vascular function and morphology in rheumatoid arthritis: a systematic review. *Rheumatology (Oxford)*. 2011;50:2125-2139.

63 Dimitroulas T, Douglas KM, Panoulas VF, et al. Derangement of hemostasis in rheumatoid arthritis: association with demographic, inflammatory and metabolic factors. *Clin Rheumatol*. 2013;32:1357-1364.

64 Prati C, Demougeot C, Guillot X, Godfrin-Valnet M, Wendling D. Endothelial dysfunction in joint disease. *Joint Bone Spine*. 2014;81:386-391.

Chapter 4

Cardiovascular disease risk evaluation

Silvia Rollefstad, Cynthia S Crowson, Piet van Riel, and
Anne Grete Semb

Screening for and diagnostics of cardiovascular disease in rheumatoid arthritis

Several studies have shown that the cardiovascular disease (CVD) risk
in patients with rheumatoid arthritis (RA) is underestimated [1–5]. In
part, this relates to underuse of tools for systematic evaluation of CVD
risk and prevention. Management of CVD risk in patients with RA is an
interdisciplinary task, and there is confusion about which health care
providers should be responsible for recording and evaluating CVD risk
factors, modifying lifestyle-related risk factors, and initiating appropriate preventive measures. Whether performance of CVD risk evaluation
should be the responsibility of the rheumatologist or other health care
providers such as general practitioners, specialists in internal medicine,
or cardiologists will probably depend on the health care system and
economic priorities in each country. However, it may be argued that the
responsibility to ensure that a CVD risk evaluation is performed should
lie with the rheumatologist as the majority of RA patients are mainly in
contact with the health care system in relation to their joint disease [1].

© Springer International Publishing Switzerland 2017
A.G. Semb (ed.), *Handbook of Cardiovascular Disease Management
in Rheumatoid Arthritis*, DOI 10.1007/978-3-319-26782-1_4

Evaluation of cardiovascular disease risk in rheumatoid arthritis

The first step in management of the high CVD risk in patients with RA is to improve CVD risk factor recording. Such recordings have been shown to be inadequate in RA, despite the increased CVD risk in this patient population [3,5]. The patients' age and sex should obviously be taken into consideration as well as medical history including smoking status, alcohol consumption, presence of chronic diseases, familial CVD, previous CVD or symptoms of CVD (ie, chest pain, dyspnea, edema, leg pain during walking), and medication use. To perform a general physical examination with specific focus on signs of hypercholesterolemia, auscultation of the large arteries, peripheral circulatory status, body height and weight, waist circumference, and blood pressure measurement is relevant. Important laboratory tests are lipid profile, fasting blood glucose/glycated hemoglobin (HbA1c), inflammatory markers (C-reactive protein [CRP] and erythrocyte sedimentation rate [ESR]), hemoglobin, liver enzymes, creatinine kinase, kidney, and thyroid function. Additional examinations may be indicated such as electrocardiogram, transthoracic echocardiography, and ultrasound of the carotid arteries. Individual CVD risk stratification performed using the Systematic COronary Risk Evaluation (SCORE) model is recommended in Europe. Other risk calculators are developed and available for use in different countries around the world. These will be described later in the chapter in the section on CVD risk calculators on page 57. An example of how to perform a CVD risk evaluation in patients with RA is illustrated in Figure 4.1.

Challenges during cardiovascular disease risk evaluation of rheumatoid arthritis patients

Several factors complicate the evaluation of CVD risk in RA patients. CVD risk calculators developed for the general population (SCORE, Framingham, Reynolds, and QRESEARCH Cardiovascular Risk Algorithm [QRISK] 2) have been reported to inaccurately predict the risk of future CVD events in patients with RA [6,7], which is elucidated in detail later on in this chapter. The imprecise estimation of CVD risk may be due to low lipid levels confounded by systemic inflammation (Figure 4.2), the female preponderance of RA patients, and the high frequency of asymptomatic atherosclerosis [8–11], which is not taken into account when the CVD risk evaluation is only based on estimated CVD risk by the SCORE CVD risk calculator [12], or other related risk prediction algorithms.

Several prospective studies report an association between the presence of carotid plaques (CP) and the risk for CVD events in non-RA subjects without documented CVD [13–18]. In the Atherosclerosis Risk in Communities study, which comprised 13,145 persons followed

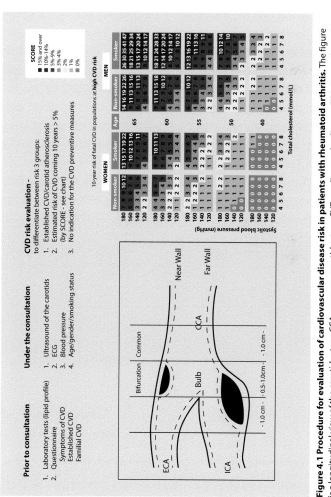

Figure 4.1 Procedure for evaluation of cardiovascular disease risk in patients with rheumatoid arthritis. The figure is a longitudinal view of the carotid artery. CCA, common carotid artery; CVD, cardiovascular disease; ECA, External carotid artery; ECG, electrocardiogram; ICA, Internal carotid artery; SCORE, Systematic COronary Risk Evaluation. Adapted from © Elsevier. All rights reserved. Perk et al [22]. Adapted from © John Wiley and Sons. All rights reserved. Del Rincon et al [23].

for approximately 16 years, it was shown that adding CP and carotid intima-media thickness (c-IMT) to the Framingham CVD risk calculator improved CVD risk prediction [19]. Approximately 23% of the patients were reclassified to a more appropriate CVD risk group by adding c-IMT and CP, and the Net Reclassification Index was 9.9%. CP are associated with poor CVD-free survival and are strongly linked to future acute coronary syndrome (ACS) in patients with RA, with a rate of ACS per 100 person years (95% confidence interval [CI]) at 1.1 (0.6, 1.7) for RA patients with no CP, and 4.3 (2.9, 6.3) for those with bilateral plaques (Figure 4.3) [20,21]. In the current European Guidelines on CVD prevention, screening for carotid artery atherosclerosis is recommended for patients at moderate CVD risk (class: IIa, level of evidence: B, and GRADE: strong) [22]. Furthermore, for the first time, autoimmune diseases such as RA, systemic lupus erythematosus, and psoriasis were acknowledged as diseases associated with increased CVD risk. Moreover, the European Atherosclerosis Society (EAS)/ European Society of Cardiology (ESC) guidelines recognize occlusive arterial disease of the lower limbs and carotid artery disease as coronary heart disease equivalent conditions, and lipid lowering therapy is recommended (class: I, level of evidence: A, GRADE: strong) [22].

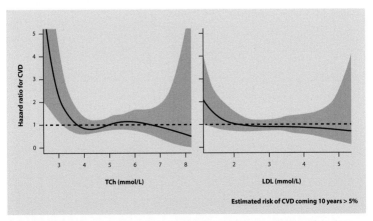

Figure 4.2 The lipid paradox in rheumatoid arthritis. Hazard ratios in solid lines. Shaded areas represent 95% confidence intervals. CVD, cardiovascular disease; LDL, low-density lipoprotein cholesterol; TCh, total cholesterol. Reproduced with permission from © BMJ Publishing Group Ltd & European League Against Rheumatism. All rights reserved. Myasoedova et al [23].

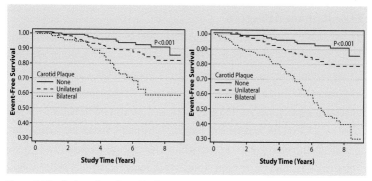

Figure 4.3 Predictive value of carotid atherosclerotic plaques regarding future acute coronary syndromes in patients with rheumatoid arthritis. Left: probability of remaining free of an initial acute coronary syndrome event among 566 patients without previous acute coronary syndrome. Right: probability of remaining free of an acute coronary syndrome event among all patients with ultrasound verified carotid plaques, n=636 (including those with previous acute coronary syndromes). Total number of events, n=121. Reproduced with permission from © John Wiley and Sons, 2011. All Rights reserved. Evans et al [20].

RA-specific factors contribute to the presence of carotid atherosclerosis in addition to traditional CVD risk factors [24]. Disease duration and disease activity have been shown to be associated with atherosclerotic plaque size and vulnerability [10,25]. Finally, ultrasound of the carotid arteries to identify atherosclerosis has been shown to reclassify a considerable proportion of RA patients into a more appropriate CVD risk group in accordance with current guidelines [22,26]. Due to the high pre-test probability for detection of carotid artery plaques by use of ultrasound in RA patients, and the clinical consequence of indication for statin treatment if a CP is present, this procedure may be added to the CVD risk evaluation for all patients with RA.

Cardiovascular disease risk calculators

CVD risk assessment for patients with RA is important, as optimal treatment of traditional CVD risk factors is crucial for reducing the risk of CVD among patients with RA. Numerous CVD risk calculators have been designed to assess the risk of CVD in the general population but their accuracy among patients with RA is questionable.

Framingham risk score

The earliest CVD risk calculator was developed in 1987 by the Framingham Heart Study [27]. A variation of this risk score was developed in 1998 and incorporated into the Third Report of the National Cholesterol Education Program (NCEP) Expert Panel on Detection, Evaluation, and Treatment of High Blood Cholesterol in Adults (Adult Treatment Panel III) – it was used as a CVD risk assessment tool in the United States for many years [28,29]. More recently the Framingham Heart Study published a new risk score with a broader CVD outcome, which included stroke, heart failure, and intermittent claudication [30]. However, the latter Framingham risk calculator was found to underestimate CVD risk among patients with RA [6,7]. Figure 4.4 demonstrates the underestimation of risk by the Framingham risk score for general CVD among patients with RA in the cohort from Olmsted County, Minnesota, USA. The treatment threshold for this risk calculator is 20% and several of the discrepancies between

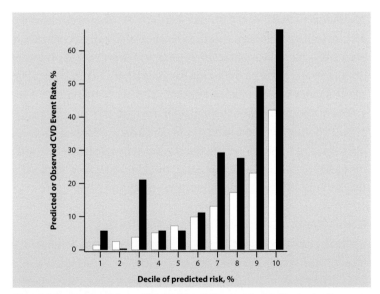

Figure 4.4 Comparison of observed and predicted 10-year risk of cardiovascular disease among patients with rheumatoid arthritis from Olmsted County, Minnesota, USA, according to deciles of predicted risk (clear bars) obtained from the Framingham risk score. The observed risk (CVD events, black bars) was obtained using Kaplan-Meier methods and is clearly higher than the predicted risk for several deciles. Reproduced with permission from © Elsevier, 2012. All Rights reserved. Crowson et al [6].

predicted and observed risks fall into this range, which means use of this risk calculator among patients with RA could lead to under-treatment with lipid lowering medications.

Reynolds Risk Score

The Reynolds risk score was also developed in the US [31,32]. It boasted improved CVD risk prediction due to the inclusion of CRP. Given the role of inflammation in the development of CVD among patients with RA, it was thought that the Reynolds risk score might perform better than the Framingham risk score for patients with RA, but this did not prove to be so [6,7].

American College of Cardiology/American Heart Association pooled cohort equation for cardiovascular disease risk evaluation

More recently, the American College of Cardiology/American Heart Association (ACC/AHA) Pooled Cohort Equation was developed and it replaced the Framingham as the risk tool of choice for CVD risk assessment in the US, despite controversy that this new risk calculator may overestimate CVD risk and consequently overrecommend statin therapy [33,34]. Improvements included in this new risk calculator compared with the Framingham risk score were the inclusion of race/ethnicity as a risk factor and the inclusion of stroke in the CVD outcome. The accuracy of prediction for this risk calculator among patients with RA has not yet been assessed.

QRISK2

In the UK, the QRISK2 was developed for CVD risk assessment [35]. It contains ethnicity, social deprivation, and other clinical conditions such as RA. While the measure of deprivation is specific to the UK, the score can be computed without this for use in other countries. The inclusion of RA in this risk score raised hopes that it would more accurately predict CVD risk for patients with RA than the other risk calculators. However, QRISK2 was found to overestimate the risk of CVD in a population-based cohort of patients with RA from the Netherlands [7].

SCORE

The SCORE calculator was developed to provide accurate CVD risk prediction in Europe [12]. It was derived from pooled data from 12 European cohort studies including >200,000 patients. A unique aspect of SCORE is that separate risk estimates were provided for high- and low-risk countries within Europe. There are now multiple country-specific versions of SCORE and the use of SCORE for CVD risk assessment is recommended by the EAS/ESC Guidelines for CVD prevention [22,36]. However, SCORE was found to generally underestimate the risk of CVD among patients with RA in the Netherlands [7].

Summary of cardiovascular disease risk factors in various risk calculators

All the risk calculators discussed thus far provided predictions of 10-year CVD risk. A summary of characteristics of these risk calculators is provided in Table 4.1 and lists of the risk factors included in each risk calculator are provided in Table 4.2.

Lifetime risk of CVD

Predicting lifetime CVD risk is also thought to be important, particularly among the often low-risk groups of the young and women [37]. Estimation of lifetime CVD risk may be more helpful to motivate lifestyle changes in these low risk groups. It may also identify patients for intervention at younger ages. Figure 4.5 demonstrates how lifetime risk might be integrated into cardiovascular risk assessments [38]. In this model diabetes mellitus and not RA was included as a separate risk factor. QRISK Lifetime was developed to estimate lifetime risk of CVD in the United Kingdom [39]. The Joint British Societies for the prevention of CVD (JBS3) recommend assessment of both 10-year and lifetime CVD risk to recognize the impact of duration of risk factors on future CVD events [40]. In the US, the CVD Lifetime Risk Pooling Project includes data from 20 community-based cohorts and was developed to study factors that influence the accurate prediction of lifetime risks [41]. The accuracy of lifetime risk assessment among patients with RA has not been evaluated.

Rheumatoid arthritis-specific risk evaluation

Given the known inaccuracies of CVD risk calculators for assessment of risk among patients with RA, the European League Against Rheumatism (EULAR) recommended use of a 1.5 multiplier to improve CVD risk prediction in RA [42]. While this was a sensible recommendation, it did not prove to increase the accuracy of risk prediction for patients with RA [6]. Since traditional CVD risk factors do not explain all the risk for CVD,

Risk calculator	Target population	CVD outcome	Applicable age range (years)	Treatment threshold (%)
Framingham risk score (Adult Treatment Panel III)	US	Hard coronary heart disease	30–74	10
Framingham risk score for general CVD	US	CVD events (fatal/non-fatal) including acute coronary syndrome (myocardial infarction, unstable angina pectoris), chronic ischemic heart disease (stable angina pectoris), coronary revascularization (percutaneous coronary intervention and coronary artery bypass grafting), coronary death, other cardiovascular death, cerebrovascular events (ischemic cerebrovascular accident and transient ischemic attack) and peripheral vascular events (non-coronary revascularization procedures, peripheral artery disease), and heart failure	30–74	20
Reynolds risk score	US	Myocardial infarction, ischemic stroke, coronary revascularization, and cardiovascular death	50+	10
ACC/AHA Pooled Cohort Equation	US	Hard atherosclerotic CVD events (defined as first occurrence of nonfatal myocardial infarction, coronary heart disease death, or fatal or nonfatal stroke)	40–79	7.5
QRISK2	UK	Coronary heart disease, stroke, and transient ischaemic attack	35–74	10
SCORE	EU	Fatal CVD events	40–65	5

Table 4.1 Characteristics of 10-year cardiovascular disease risk calculators designed for use in the general population. ACC/AHA, American College of Cardiology/American Heart Association; CVD, cardiovascular disease; QRISK, QRESEARCH Cardiovascular Risk Algorithm; SCORE, Systematic COronary Risk Evaluation.

as noted in Chapter 3, researchers advocated for a CVD risk calculator designed specifically for patients with RA, which would incorporate measures of inflammation and RA disease characteristics [4]. The Expanded Cardiovascular Risk Prediction Score for Rheumatoid Arthritis (ERS-RA) was recently developed for this purpose [43]. This CVD risk algorithm

	Framingham risk score (Adult Treatment Panel III)	Framingham risk score for general CVD	Reynolds risk score	ACC/AHA pooled cohort equation	QRISK2	SCORE
Age/sex	✓	✓	✓	✓	✓	✓
Postcode					✓	
Race/Ethnicity				✓	✓	
Body mass index					✓	
Smoking	✓	✓	✓	✓	✓	✓
Family history of premature coronary heart disease			✓		✓	
Diastolic blood pressure	✓					
Systolic blood pressure	✓	✓	✓	✓		✓
Anti-hypertensive use	✓	✓		✓		
Total cholesterol	✓	✓	✓	✓	✓	✓
High density lipoprotein	✓	✓	✓	✓	✓	✓
Diabetes mellitus	✓	✓	✓		✓	
Hemoglobin A_{1c} for diabetics			✓			
Rheumatoid arthritis					✓	
Atrial fibrillation					✓	
Chronic kidney disease					✓	
High sensitivity C-reactive protein			✓			

Table 4.2 Risk factor data required for calculation of 10-year cardiovascular disease risk calculators designed for use in the general population. ACC, American College of Cardiology; AHA, American Heart Association; CVD, cardiovascular disease; QRISK, QRESEARCH Cardiovascular Risk Algorithm; SCORE, Systematic COronary Risk Evaluation.

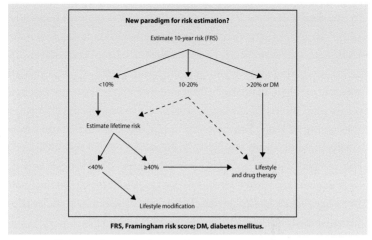

Figure 4.5 Lifetime cardiovascular disease risk assessment. Illustration of how lifetime risk assessment might be incorporated into cardiovascular risk assessment to provide earlier identification and treatment of younger patients with high lifetime risks. DM, diabetes mellitus; FRD, Framingham risk score. Reproduced with permission from © Wolters Kluwer Health, Inc, 2006. All rights reserved. Lloyd-Jones et al [22].

includes additional RA disease characteristics including the Clinical Disease Activity Index, Health Assessment Questionnaire Disability Index, use of corticosteroids and RA disease duration [44,45]. However, the ERS-RA risk calculator has many limitations including the lack of key CVD risk factors, such as blood pressure (BP) and lipids. It relies instead on the physician's diagnoses of hypertension and dyslipidemia, both of which are known to be under-diagnosed among patients with RA [46,47]. Caution is warranted because an external validation is needed before clinical adoption of this CVD risk calculator should be considered. It is unclear whether this risk calculator improves CVD risk prediction in patients with RA enough to warrant the additional time needed to calculate it [48].

Cardiovascular disease prevention

Lipids

To decide if there is indication for lipid lowering treatment in apparently healthy persons, one should evaluate the total burden of CVD risk factors. The SCORE CVD risk calculator (Figure 4.1) is recommended by the EAS/ESC for CVD risk evaluation in the general population [22]. The SCORE algorithm incorporates traditional risk factors for CVD: age, sex, systolic BP, cholesterol values (total cholesterol [TC] or TC and high-density lipoprotein cholesterol [HDL-c]), and smoking status to estimate the risk of a fatal atherosclerotic event (for example, myocardial infarction, ischemic stroke, and aneurysm of the aorta) in the coming 10 years. The cut off values for initiation of CVD preventive treatment with statins are shown in Figure 4.6. Use of the SCORE CVD risk calculator yields an absolute risk estimate, however this may not be adequate for younger persons with a low absolute risk, but high relative risk of CVD. A relative risk chart is developed to help advise these persons regarding lifestyle interventions (Figure 4.7).

Definitions of primary and secondary prevention

Primary prevention

For patients without established CVD with a calculated CVD risk by SCORE of 5% or greater (10-year risk of a fatal atherosclerotic event), lipid-lowering treatment is indicated. Low HDL-c and high triglyceride levels are described as markers of increased risk, but there is not sufficient evidence to consider any specific levels of HDL-c and triglycerides as recommended treatment targets according to the ESC guidelines [22]. However, the recommended levels of triglycerides and HDL-c are ≤1.7 mmol/L and ≥1.0/1.2 mmol/L (males/females), respectively, both for primary and secondary prevention purposes.

Secondary prevention

Patients in the very high risk group are, according to the latest EAS/ESC guidelines for CVD prevention [22], those with documented CVD by invasive or non-invasive testing (such as coronary angiography or CP on ultrasound), previous myocardial infarction, ACS, coronary/arterial revascularization, ischemic stroke, peripheral artery disease, diabetes mellitus with one or more CVD risk factors and/or target organ damage, and patients with severe chronic kidney disease. A calculated CVD risk by SCORE of 10% or greater also indicates a very high risk of CVD. These patients should have the highest priority for treatment, and the recommended lipid targets are lower. If the

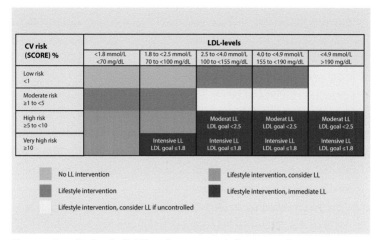

Figure 4.6 Cut-off values for lipid lowering treatment indication. Lipid lowering treatment indication relies both on the 10-year risk estimate of fatal cardiovascular disease and low-density lipoprotein cholesterol levels. CV, cardiovascular; LDL, low density lipoprotein; LL, lipid lowering; SCORE, Systematic COronary Risk Evaluation. Adapted from © Elsevier. All rights reserved. Perk et al [22].

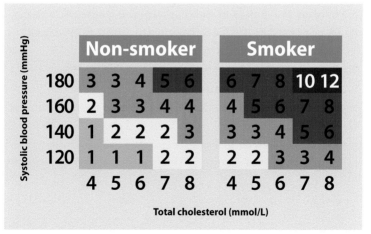

Figure 4.7 Relative risk chart for 10-year mortality. This relative risk chart is recommended for use in young persons. A person in the upper box at the right hand has a 12-time higher 10-year mortality risk compared to a person in the bottom left box. Reproduced with permission from © Elsevier. All rights reserved. Perk et al [22].

low density lipoprotein cholesterol (LDL-c) goal is not possible to obtain, a 50% or greater reduction from baseline LDL-c is considered at target level.

Blood pressure/hypertension

Hypertension seems to be both underdiagnosed and undertreated in patients with RA [49–51]. It is a major modifiable risk factor for CVD, and BP should be regularly monitored in patients with RA. Measurement of BP at the upper arm is recommended, and cuff and bladder size should fit the dimension of the arm. To perform a correct BP measurement the following stages are recommended [52]:

1. The patient should rest for 3–5 minutes before BP recording.
2. At least 2 measurements should be taken approximately 1–2 minutes apart. Additional measurements may be performed if the two first differ significantly (>5 mmHg). Calculate the average BP of the measurements considered appropriate.
3. In patients with arrhythmias, repeated measurements are recommended to increase accuracy.
4. The cuff should be placed at the heart level.
5. At first visit, BP measurements in both arms may be performed.
6. In elderly and in diabetic patients, measurement of orthostatic hypotension is indicated.
7. If suspicion of white coat hypertension, ambulatory BP measurement may be considered.

BP categories are displayed in Table 4.3. Indication for antihypertensive treatment should be decided on the basis of the total CVD risk for each patient, and not solely on BP levels. The current recommendations regarding

Category	Systolic		Diastolic
Optimal	<120	and	<80
Normal	120–129	and/or	80–84
High normal	130–139	and/or	85–89
Grade 1 hypertension	140–159	and/or	90–99
Grade 2 hypertension	160–179	and/or	100–109
Grade 3 hypertension	≥180	and/or	≥110
Isolated systolic hypertension	≥140	and	<90

Table 4.3 Blood pressure categories. Reproduced with permission from © Wolters Kluwer Health, Inc, 2013. All rights reserved. Mancia et al [52].

antihypertensive treatment indication and BP goals for the general population are summarized in Figure 4.8. Whether these anti-hypertensives and BP goals are optimal for patients with RA is not known. Several risk factors besides BP are of interest in the total CVD risk evaluation, they are [52]:

- Male sex
- Age (men ≥55 years; women ≥65 years

Other risk factors, asymptomatic organ damage or disease	Blood Pressure (mmHg)			
	High normal SBP 130-139 or DBP 85-89	Grade 1 HT SBP 140-159 or DBP 90-99	Grade 2 HT SBP 160-179 or DBP 100-109	Grade 3 HT SBP ≥180 or DBP ≥110
No other RF	• No BP intervention	• Lifestyle changes for several months • Then add BP drugs targeting <140/90	• Lifestyle changes for several weeks • Then add BP drugs targeting <140/90	• Lifestyle changes • Immediate BP drugs targeting <140/90
1-2 RF	• Lifestyle changes • No BP intervention	• Lifestyle changes for several weeks • Then add BP drugs targeting <140/90	• Lifestyle changes for several weeks • Then add BP drugs targeting <140/90	• Lifestyle changes • Immediate BP drugs targeting <140/90
≥3 RF	• Lifestyle changes • No BP intervention	• Lifestyle changes for several weeks • Then add BP drugs targeting <140/90	• Lifestyle changes • BP drugs targeting <140/90	• Lifestyle changes • Immediate BP drugs targeting <140/90
OD, CKD stage 3 or diabetes	• Lifestyle changes • No BP intervention	• Lifestyle changes • BP drugs targeting <140/90	• Lifestyle changes • BP drugs targeting <140/90	• Lifestyle changes • Immediate BP drugs targeting <140/90
Symptomatic CVD, CKD stage ≥4 or diabetes with OD/RFs	• Lifestyle changes • No BP intervention	• Lifestyle changes • BP drugs targeting <140/90	• Lifestyle changes • BP drugs targeting <140/90	• Lifestyle changes • Immediate BP drugs targeting <140/90

Figure 4.8 Antihypertensive treatment indications. BR, blood pressure; CKD, chronic kidney disease DBP, diastolic blood pressure; HT, hypertension; OD, organ damage; RF, risk factor; SBP, systolic blood pressure. Reproduced with permission from ©Wolters Kluwer Health, Inc, 2013. All rights reserved. Mancia et al [52].

- Dyslipidemia:
  - Total cholesterol >4.9 mmol/L (190 mg/dL), and/or
  - Low-density lipoprotein cholesterol >3.0 mmol/L (115 mg/dL), and/or
  - High-density lipoprotein cholesterol: men <1.0 mmol/L (40 mg/dL), women <1.2 mmol/L (46 mg/dL), and/or
  - Triglycerides >1.7 mmol/L (150 mg/dL)
- Fasting plasma glucose 5.6–6.9 mmol/L (102–125 mg/dL)
- Abnormal glucose tolerance test
- Obesity (body mass index $\geq$30 kg/m^2)
- Abdominal obesity (waist circumference: men $\geq$102 cm; women $\geq$88 cm; in Caucasians)
- Family history of premature cardiovascular disease (men <55 years of age; women <65 years of age)

Diabetes mellitus

The CVD risk in patients with concomitant diagnoses of RA and diabetes mellitus seems to be additive [53], and these patients need special attention regarding CVD preventive measures. However, no treatment guidelines exist for this specific patient population. In the 2012 EAS/ESC guidelines for CVD prevention for the general population the following is recommended [22]:

1. HbA1c target is <7%, but hypoglycemia and weight gain must be avoided, and individual approaches must be considered in patients with complex disease.
2. Statins are recommended for primary prevention purposes in patients with Type 1 diabetes mellitus with target organ damage and for all patients with Type 2 diabetes mellitus.
3. Metformin should be used as first-line therapy in patients with Type 2 diabetes mellitus.
4. A BP target of <140/80 mmHg is recommended.
5. Antiplatelet therapy is not recommended solely on the basis of a diabetes mellitus diagnosis.

References

1   Bell C, Rowe IF. The recognition and assessment of cardiovascular risk in people with rheumatoid arthritis in primary care: a questionnaire-based study of general practitioners. *Musculoskeletal Care*. 2011;9:69-74.

2   Bartels CM, Kind AJ, Thorpe CT, et al. Lipid testing in patients with rheumatoid arthritis and key cardiovascular-related comorbidities: a medicare analysis. *Semin Arthritis Rheum*. 2012;42:9-16.

3   Ikdahl E, Rollefstad S, Olsen IC, et al. EULAR task force recommendations on annual cardiovascular risk assessment for patients with rheumatoid arthritis: an audit of the success of implementation in a rheumatology outpatient clinic. *Biomed Res Int*. 2015;2015:515280.

4   Crowson CS, Gabriel SE. Towards improving cardiovascular risk management in patients with rheumatoid arthritis: the need for accurate risk assessment. *Ann Rheum Dis*. 2011;70:719-721.

5   Teir J, Koduri G, Meadows A, et al. An audit of recording cardiovascular risk factors in patients with rheumatoid arthritis and systemic lupus erythematosus in centres in East Anglia and the South East. *Rheumatology (Oxford)*. 2008;47:1252-1254.

6   Crowson CS, Matteson EL, Roger VL, Therneau TM, Gabriel SE. Usefulness of risk scores to estimate the risk of cardiovascular disease in patients with rheumatoid arthritis. *Am J Cardiol*. 2012;110:420-424.

7   Arts EE, Popa C, den Broeder AA, et al. Performance of four current risk algorithms in predicting cardiovascular events in patients with early rheumatoid arthritis. *Ann Rheum Dis*. 2015;74:668-674.

8   Roman MJ, Moeller E, Davis A, et al. Preclinical carotid atherosclerosis in patients with rheumatoid arthritis. *Ann Intern Med*. 2006;144:249-256.

9   Kobayashi H, Giles JT, Polak JF, et al. Increased prevalence of carotid artery atherosclerosis in rheumatoid arthritis is artery-specific. *J Rheumatol*. 2010;37:730-739.

10 Semb AG, Rollefstad S, Provan SA et al. Carotid plaque characteristics and disease activity in rheumatoid arthritis. *J Rheumatol*. 2013;40:359-368.

11 Ambrosino P, Lupoli R, Di MA, Tasso M, Peluso R, Di Minno MN. Subclinical atherosclerosis in patients with rheumatoid arthritis. A meta-analysis of literature studies. *Thromb Haemost*. 2015;113:916-930.

12 Conroy RM, Pyorala K, Fitzgerald AP, et al. Estimation of ten-year risk of fatal cardiovascular disease in Europe: the SCORE project. *Eur Heart J*. 2003;24:987-1003.

13 Kitamura A, Iso H, Imano H, et al. Carotid intima-media thickness and plaque characteristics as a risk factor for stroke in Japanese elderly men. *Stroke*. 2004;35:2788-2794.

14 Rosvall M, Janzon L, Berglund G, Engstrom G, Hedblad B. Incident coronary events and case fatality in relation to common carotid intima-media thickness. *J Intern Med*. 2005;257:430-437.

15 van der Meer IM, Bots ML, Hofman A, del Sol AI, van der Kuip DA, Witteman JC. Predictive value of noninvasive measures of atherosclerosis for incident myocardial infarction: the Rotterdam Study. *Circulation*. 2004;109:1089-1094.

16 Salonen JT, Salonen R. Ultrasonographically assessed carotid morphology and the risk of coronary heart disease. *Arterioscler Thromb*. 1991;11:1245-1249.

17 Prabhakaran S, Rundek T, Ramas R, et al. Carotid plaque surface irregularity predicts ischemic stroke: the northern Manhattan study. *Stroke*. 2006;37:2696-2701.

18 Hunt KJ, Sharrett AR, Chambless LE, Folsom AR, Evans GW, Heiss G. Acoustic shadowing on B-mode ultrasound of the carotid artery predicts CHD. *Ultrasound Med Biol*. 2001;27:357-365.

19 Nambi V, Chambless L, Folsom AR, et al. Carotid intima-media thickness and presence or absence of plaque improves prediction of coronary heart disease risk: the ARIC (Atherosclerosis Risk In Communities) study. *J Am Coll Cardiol*. 2010;55:1600-1607.

20 Evans MR, Escalante A, Battafarano DF, Freeman GL, O'Leary DH, del Rincón I. Carotid atherosclerosis predicts incident acute coronary syndromes in rheumatoid arthritis. *Arthritis Rheum*. 2011;63:1211-1220.

21 Ajeganova S, de FU, Jogestrand T, Frostegard J, Hafstrom I. Carotid atherosclerosis, disease measures, oxidized low-density lipoproteins, and atheroprotective natural antibodies for cardiovascular disease in early rheumatoid arthritis -- an inception cohort study. *J Rheumatol.* 2012;39:1146-1154.

22 Perk J, De BG, Gohlke H, et al. European Guidelines on cardiovascular disease prevention in clinical practice (version 2012): The Fifth Joint Task Force of the European Society of Cardiology and Other Societies on Cardiovascular Disease Prevention in Clinical Practice (constituted by representatives of nine societies and by invited experts). *Atherosclerosis.* 2012;223:1-68.

23 Myasoedova E. Lipid paradox in rheumatoid arthritus: the impact of serum lipid measures and systemic inflammation on the risk of cardiovascular disease. *Ann Rheum Dis.* 2011;70:482-487.

24 del Rincon I, Freeman GL, Haas RW, O'Leary DH, Escalante A. Relative contribution of cardiovascular risk factors and rheumatoid arthritis clinical manifestations to atherosclerosis. *Arthritis Rheum.* 2005;52:3413-3423.

25 Wallberg-Jonsson S, Ohman M, Rantapaa-Dahlqvist S. Which factors are related to the presence of atherosclerosis in rheumatoid arthritis? *Scand J Rheumatol.* 2004;33:373-379.

26 Corrales A, Gonzalez-Juanatey C, Peiro ME, Blanco R, Llorca J, Gonzalez-Gay MA. Carotid ultrasound is useful for the cardiovascular risk stratification of patients with rheumatoid arthritis: results of a population-based study. *Ann Rheum Dis.* 2014;73:722-727.

27 Wilson PW, Castelli WP, Kannel WB. Coronary risk prediction in adults (the Framingham Heart Study). *Am J Cardiol.* 1987;59:91G-94G.

28 National Cholesterol Education Program (NCEP) Expert Panel on Detection, Evaluation, and Treatment of High Blood Cholesterol in Adults (Adult Treatment Panel III).Third Report of the National Cholesterol Education Program (NCEP) Expert Panel on Detection, Evaluation, and Treatment of High Blood Cholesterol in Adults (Adult Treatment Panel III) final report. *Circulation.* 2002;106:3143-3421.

29 Wilson PW, d'Agostino RB, Levy D, Belanger AM, Silbershatz H, Kannel WB. Prediction of coronary heart disease using risk factor categories. *Circulation.* 1998;97:1837-1847.

30 D'Agostino RB, Sr., Vasan RS, Pencina MJ et al. General cardiovascular risk profile for use in primary care: the Framingham Heart Study. *Circulation.* 2008;117:743-753.

31 Ridker PM, Buring JE, Rifai N, Cook NR. Development and validation of improved algorithms for the assessment of global cardiovascular risk in women: the Reynolds Risk Score. *JAMA.* 2007;297:611-619.

32 Ridker PM, Paynter NP, Rifai N, Gaziano JM, Cook NR. C-reactive protein and parental history improve global cardiovascular risk prediction: the Reynolds Risk Score for men. *Circulation.* 2008;118:2243-2251.

33 Goff DC Jr, Lloyd-Jones DM, Bennett G, et al. 2013 ACC/AHA guideline on the assessment of cardiovascular risk: a report of the American College of Cardiology/American Heart Association Task Force on Practice Guidelines. *J Am Coll Cardiol.* 2014;63:2935-2959.

34 Ridker PM, Cook NR. Statins: new American guidelines for prevention of cardiovascular disease. *Lancet.* 2013;382:1762-1765.

35 Hippisley-Cox J, Coupland C, Vinogradova Y, et al. Predicting cardiovascular risk in England and Wales: prospective derivation and validation of QRISK2. *BMJ.* 2008;336:1475-1482.

36 Catapano AL, Chapman J, Wiklund O, Taskinen MR. The new joint EAS/ESC guidelines for the management of dyslipidaemias. *Atherosclerosis.* 2011;217:1.

37 Lloyd-Jones DM, Larson MG, Beiser A, Levy D. Lifetime risk of developing coronary heart disease. *Lancet.* 1999;353:89-92.

38 Lloyd-Jones DM. Short-term versus long-term risk for coronary artery disease: implications for lipid guidelines. *Curr Opin Lipidol.* 2006;17:619-625.

39 Hippisley-Cox J, Coupland C, Robson J, Brindle P. Derivation, validation, and evaluation of a new QRISK model to estimate lifetime risk of cardiovascular disease: cohort study using QResearch database. *BMJ.* 2010;341:c6624.

40 JBS3 Board. Joint British Societies' consensus recommendations for the prevention of cardiovascular disease (JBS3). *Heart*. 2014;100:ii1-ii67.

41 Wilkins JT, Karmali KN, Huffman MD, et al. Data Resource Profile: The Cardiovascular Disease Lifetime Risk Pooling Project. *Int J Epidemiol*. 2015;44:1557-1564.

42 Peters MJ, Symmons DP, McCarey D, et al. EULAR evidence-based recommendations for cardiovascular risk management in patients with rheumatoid arthritis and other forms of inflammatory arthritis. *Ann Rheum Dis*. 2010;69:325-331.

43 Solomon DH, Greenberg J, Curtis JR, et al. Derivation and internal validation of an expanded cardiovascular risk prediction score for rheumatoid arthritis: a Consortium of Rheumatology Researchers of North America Registry Study. *Arthritis Rheumatol*. 2015;67:1995-2003.

44 Aletaha D, Nell VP, Stamm T, et al. Acute phase reactants add little to composite disease activity indices for rheumatoid arthritis: validation of a clinical activity score. *Arthritis Res Ther*. 2005;7:R796-R806.

45 Pincus T, Summey JA, Soraci SA Jr, Wallston KA, Hummon NP. Assessment of patient satisfaction in activities of daily living using a modified Stanford Health Assessment Questionnaire. *Arthritis Rheum*. 1983;26:1346-1353.

46 Panoulas VF, Douglas KM, Milionis HJ, et al. Prevalence and associations of hypertension and its control in patients with rheumatoid arthritis. *Rheumatology (Oxford)*. 2007;46:1477-1482.

47 Toms TE, Panoulas VF, Douglas KM, et al. Statin use in rheumatoid arthritis in relation to actual cardiovascular risk: evidence for substantial undertreatment of lipid-associated cardiovascular risk? *Ann Rheum Dis*. 2010;69:683-688.

48 Symmons DP. Do we need a disease-specific cardiovascular risk calculator for patients with rheumatoid arthritis? *Arthritis Rheumatol*. 2015;67:1990-1994.

49 Han C, Robinson DW Jr, Hackett MV, Paramore LC, Fraeman KH, Bala MV. Cardiovascular disease and risk factors in patients with rheumatoid arthritis, psoriatic arthritis, and ankylosing spondylitis. *J Rheumatol*. 2006;33:2167-2172.

50 Panoulas VF, Metsios GS, Pace AV, et al. Hypertension in rheumatoid arthritis. *Rheumatology (Oxford)*. 2008;47:1286-1298.

51 Bartels CM, Johnson H, Voelker K, et al. Impact of rheumatoid arthritis on receiving a diagnosis of hypertension among patients with regular primary care. *Arthritis Care Res (Hoboken)*. 2014;66:1281-1288.

52 Mancia G, Fagard R, Narkiewicz K, et al. 2013 ESH/ESC Guidelines for the management of arterial hypertension: the Task Force for the management of arterial hypertension of the European Society of Hypertension (ESH) and of the European Society of Cardiology (ESC). *J Hypertens*. 2013;31:1281-1357.

53 Lindhardsen J, Ahlehoff O, Gislason GH, et al. The risk of myocardial infarction in rheumatoid arthritis and diabetes mellitus: a Danish nationwide cohort study. *Ann Rheum Dis*. 2011;70:929-934.

Chapter 5

Pharmacological management of cardiovascular disease in patients with rheumatoid arthritis

Silvia Rollefstad, Eirik Ikdahl, and Anne Grete Semb

Introduction

Although there is a large body of knowledge on the increased cardiovascular disease (CVD) risk in rheumatoid arthritis (RA), there is a lack of clinical evidence on management of the increased risk.

Current treatment recommendations

Several treatment guidelines exist regarding prevention of CVD for the general population, including both national guidelines and guidelines for larger geographical areas such as Europe and US. In the latest European Society of Cardiology (ESC) guidelines for CVD prevention, the presence of RA was mentioned as a high CVD risk factor for the first time [1]. However, an RA diagnosis itself should not be considered as an indication for initiation of cardio-protective treatment, but is recommended to be taken into consideration when evaluating the total CVD risk for each patient.

European League Against Rheumatism recommendations

A task force of the European League Against Rheumatism (EULAR) published recommendations in 2010 regarding management of CVD risk in patients with RA and other inflammatory joint diseases [2]. These

© Springer International Publishing Switzerland 2017
A.G. Semb (ed.), *Handbook of Cardiovascular Disease Management in Rheumatoid Arthritis*, DOI 10.1007/978-3-319-26782-1_5

recommendations suggested that in RA patients fulfilling at least two out of three of specified criteria (disease duration >10 years, rheumatoid factor/anticitrullinated protein antibody positivity, or extra-articular manifestations), the calculated CVD risk should be multiplied by 1.5. This multiplication factor was derived mainly from relevant standardized mortality ratios because information from large-scale prospective cohort studies was, and still is, lacking. However, Corrales et al have shown that the discussed multiplication factor only reclassifies 3% of the patients into more appropriate CVD risk classes, but even then patients at high CVD risk and those with asymptomatic carotid atherosclerosis were not adequately identified. Hence, the 1.5 multiplication factor does not fully account for the increased risk of CVD in RA [3].

The EULAR recommendations were updated in 2015, and include several new recommendations [4], which were presented at the annual EULAR conference in 2015, and will be published in 2016. A CVD risk assessment is currently recommended to be performed at least every five years, as no evidence supports that yearly screening reduces CVD morbidity and mortality in RA patients. National guidelines developed for the general population should be followed with respect to CVD risk estimation. If no national guidelines are available, use of the Systematic COronary Risk Evaluation (SCORE) CVD risk calculator is recommended. The total cholesterol (TC) and high-density lipoprotein cholesterol (HDL-c) is preferred over use of only TC levels to estimate future CVD risk in RA patients. It was decided that the 1.5 multiplication factor should still be recommended to be used during CVD risk evaluation, but now for all RA patients. A new recommendation includes that screening for asymptomatic atherosclerotic plaques by use of carotid ultrasound may be considered as part of the CVD risk evaluation in patients with RA. The importance of a healthy diet, regular exercise, and smoking cessation was emphasized. Furthermore, statins and antihypertensive treatment may be used as in the general population. Regarding anti-rheumatic treatment, optimal control of disease activity is advocated in order to reduce systemic inflammation. However, prescription of non-steroidal anti-inflammatory drugs (NSAIDs) and corticosteroids should be done with caution.

Pharmacological cardio-protective treatment in patients with rheumatoid arthritis

Anti-hypertensive treatment

Hypertension (HT) is a modifiable risk factor contributing to the increased CVD risk in patients with RA [5]. Several mechanisms may lead to the development of HT including use of certain anti-rheumatic drugs, such as corticosteroids [6], NSAIDs [7], cyclosporine [8], and leflunomide [9]. HT is associated with the presence of subclinical atherosclerosis [10], and higher BP levels have also been shown to be the most influential risk factor for arterial stiffening in RA patients [11]. For the management of HT, there is no evidence that preferred drugs or treatment thresholds should differ in patients with RA compared to the general population. Regarding the choice of antihypertensive drugs, evidence supports that the benefit of the treatment seems to be related to the lowering of the BP, and not to the specific drug used to reach this target. The 2013 ESH/ESC Guidelines for the management of arterial hypertension recommend diuretics, beta-blockers, calcium antagonists, angiotensin-converting enzyme inhibitors, and angiotensin receptor blockers as suitable options for first-line treatment of HT [12]. These medications may be given as monotherapy or in combination. However, the different antihypertensive drug classes vary in the adverse effect profile, and the drug of choice and BP treatment targets will depend on the specific condition (Table 5.1 and 5.2).

Lipid lowering medication

Statins are well established as the drug of choice to decrease cholesterol levels [1,13]. Hydroxymethylglutaryl-coenzyme A (HMG-CoA) is the precursor for cholesterol synthesis in the liver. Statins are HMG-CoA reductase inhibitors, resulting in reduced production of cholesterol, which leads to an upregulation of low-density lipoprotein cholesterol (LDL-c) receptors on the cell surface of the hepatocytes, with the consequence of increased LDL-c extraction from the blood. It is beyond all reasonable doubt that statins have a cardio-protective effect, both in primary and secondary prevention of CVD [14-16]. Furthermore, statins are generally well tolerated. The risk of myopathy is low (1/1000), but myopathy may in rare cases lead to rhabdomyolysis and renal failure. If the patients experience myalgia with no increase in creatine kinase (CK; occurs in 5–10% of treated patients), statin treatment can be continued if the muscle pain is tolerable for the patient. An elevation of CK <5 times upper limit of normal (ULN) in two blood samples is considered acceptable. Elevated liver enzymes (alanine aminotransferase and aspartate aminotransferase) occur in 0.5–2.0% of patients treated with statins, and this adverse event is dose dependent. If the increase in liver enzymes exceeds three times ULN it is recommended to discontinue the statin treatment. A small increase in incident Type 2 diabetes mellitus in statin-treated patients has been reported [17], but the CVD benefit has been shown to surpass the risk of diabetes in patients at high risk of CVD [18]. The diabetes risk for statin-treated patients were mainly in those with impaired fasting blood glucose and other major risk

Condition	Drug
Asymptomatic organ damage:	
• LVH	• ACE inhibitor, calcium antagonist, ARB
• Asymptomatic atherosclerosis	• Calcium antagonist, ACE inhibitor
• Microalbuminuria	• ACE inhibitor, ARB
• Renal dysfunction	• ACE inhibitor, ARB
Clinical CV event:	
• Previous stroke	• Any agent effectively lowering BP
• Previous myocardial infarction	• BB, ACE inhbitor, ARB
• Angina pectoris	• BB, calcium antagonist
• Heart failure	• Diuretic, BB, ACE inhibitor, ARB, mineralocorticoid receptor antagonists
• Aortic aneurysm	• BB
• Atrial fibrillation, prevention	• Consider ARB, ACE inhbitor, BB, or mineralocorticoid receptor antagonists
• Atrial fibrillation, ventricular rate control	• BB, non-dihydropyridine calcium antagonist
• ESRD/proteinuria	• ACE inhibitor, ARB
• Peripheral artery disease	• ACE inhibitor, calcium antagonist
Other risk factors in certain populations:	
• ISH (elderly)	• Diuretic, calcium antagonist
• Metabolic syndrome	• ACE inhibitor, ARB, calcium antagonist
• Diabetes mellitus	• ACE inhibitor, ARB
• Pregnancy	• Methyldopa, BB, calcium antagonist
• Black	• Diuretic, calcium antagonists

Table 5.1 Anti-hypertensive drugs for various conditions. ACE, angiotensin-converting enzyme; ARB, angiotensin receptor blocker; BB, beta-blocker; BP, blood pressure; CV, cardiovascular; ESRD, end-stage renal disease; ISH, isolated systolic hypertension; LVH, left ventricular hypertrophy. Reproduced with permission from © Wolters Kluwer Health, Inc, 2013. All rights reserved. Mancia et al [12].

factors for diabetes in the Justification for the Use of statins in primary Prevention: an Intervention Trial Evaluating Rosuvastatin (JUPITER) trial [19]. The metabolism of statins is predominantly in the liver via the cytochrome P450 system (except pravastatin, rosuvastatin, and pitavastatin). Thus, statins interact with other drugs that are metabolized through the same system. Other contraindications for statin treatment are liver disease and myopathy. Combined statin-fibrate (especially gemfibrozil) therapy is shown to increase the risk for rhabdomyolysis, and is not recommended [20]. There has been some uncertainties related to cancer and statin use, but Alsheikh-Ali et al did not find a relation of statin use and development of cancer in a meta-analyses of 15 large randomized statin trials including 437,017 person-years and 5752 cases of cancer [21]. The relation of statins and cancer development in patients with RA needs further investigation.

The level of LDL-c has been used as a response indicator in almost all trials investigating the effect of lipid-lowering therapy. A 1.0 mmol/L reduction in LDL-c is associated with a 22% reduction in CVD morbidity

Recommendations	Class[a]	Level[b]
A SBP goal <140mmHg:		
a. is recommended in patients at low–moderate CV risk;		
b. is recommended in patients with diabetes;		
c. should be considered in patients with previous stroke or TIA;		
d. should be considered in patients with CHD; and		
e. should be considered in patients with diabetic or non-diabetic CKD.		
In elderly hypertensives less than 80 years old with SBP ≥160 mmHg there is solid evidence to recommend reducing SBP to between 150 and 140 mmHg.		
In fit elderly patients less than 80 years old SBP values <140 mmHg may be considered, whereas in the fragile population SBP goals should be adapted to individual tolerability.		
In individuals older than 80 years and with initial SBP ≥160 mmHg, it is recommended to reduce SBP to between 150 and 140 mmHg provided they are in good physical and metal conditions.		
A DBP target of <90 mmHg is always recommended, except in patients with diabetes, in whom values <85 mmHg are recommended. It should nevertheless be considered that DBP values between 80 and 85 mmHg are safe and well tolerated.		

Table 5.2 Guideline recommended blood pressure targets. CHD, coronary heart disease; CKD, chronic kidney disease; CV, cardiovascular; DBP, diastolic blood pressure; SBP, systolic blood pressure; TIA, transient ischemic attack. Reproduced with permission from ©Wolters Kluwer Health, Inc, 2013. All rights reserved. Mancia et al [12].

and mortality [14]. Therefore, LDL-c is considered the major target for lipid-lowering therapy.

It has been reported that lipids are less frequently tested in patients with RA than in the general population [22]. The interaction between lipid values and inflammation [23] may indicate a need for a tighter follow-up or frequent lipid monitoring in patients with RA, although this is still an area of uncertainty. Soubrier and colleagues evaluated the prevalence of patients with RA in whom lowering LDL-c should be considered in accordance with the Adult Treatment Panel III (ATPIII) guidelines, and concluded that lipid lowering therapy was insufficiently prescribed in this patient group [24]. A significant underuse of statins for primary prevention purposes in RA patients has been reported [22,25], and the degree of under-treatment was dependent on the risk stratification method. Even after suffering a myocardial infarction, patients with RA seem to receive less CVD preventive treatment than patients without RA [26]. In addition, statin discontinuation in patients with RA has also been associated with an increased risk of death from CVD and all-cause mortality, and provides support for the importance of statin compliance in RA patients where such medication is indicated [27].

Statins are reported to have beneficial effects on the joint disease in addition to the lipid-lowering effect and reduction of CVD events. A placebo-controlled study with atorvastatin versus placebo in 116 patients with active RA revealed a significant reduction of inflammatory biomarkers, such as C-reactive protein (CRP) and erythrocyte sedimentation rate (ESR), and also a decrease in swollen joint count [28]. Reduction in RA disease activity was further confirmed in another study including 30 patients with early RA randomized to placebo or atorvastatin 40 mg daily [29]. Furthermore, statins may have favourable effects on endothelial function [29, 30], arterial stiffness [31], and on modification of HDL-c properties in patients with RA [32]. A cost-effectiveness analysis concluded that the dual effect of statins, both lipid-lowering and anti-inflammatory effects, makes this therapy cost effective in RA patients [33].

The first primary prevention trial, a randomized, placebo-controlled statin study with CVD outcome for patients with RA without diagnosed CVD, was recently presented at the American College of

Rheumatology [34]. In the TRial of Atorvastatin for the primary prevention of Cardiovascular Events in patients with Rheumatoid Arthritis (TRACE-RA), 2986 RA patients from 106 centres in the United Kingdom were randomized to atorvastatin 40 mg daily or placebo. However, due to a lower event rate than anticipated, the trial was prematurely terminated. LDL-c was significantly reduced in the atorvastatin arm compared with placebo. A 34% risk reduction for a major CVD event compared with placebo was found but this difference did not reach statistical significance, possibly due to the early termination of the trial and corresponding low number of patients and CVD events. Regarding safety, there were no differences in adverse events between the atorvastatin (19.7%) and the placebo (19.5%) group (p=0.93). Comparable results have been reported from a post hoc analysis of two large statin trials (the Incremental Decrease in Endpoints Through Aggressive Lipid lowering [IDEAL] and the Treating to New Targets [TNT] studies) in patients with coronary heart disease, which also revealed that patients with and without inflammatory joint diseases had comparable lipid-lowering effect and reduction of CVD morbidity and mortality [35].

Experiences regarding lipid lowering treatment in patients with RA have been reported from a preventive cardio-rheuma clinic. Patients with inflammatory joint diseases referred for a CVD risk evaluation from a rheumatology outpatient clinic and general practitioners in the time period 2009–12 were assessed to reveal the proportion of patients in need of CVD preventive measures [36]. Furthermore, the effects of lipid-lowering therapy were evaluated with regard to achievement of guideline-recommended lipid goals. CVD risk stratification was performed at the first consultation, and all patients received advice about physical activity and cholesterol friendly diet. Smokers were offered the opportunity to join smoking cessation programmes and diabetics were referred to a specialist clinic for optimization of glucose control if needed. Hypertensive patients were treated with antihypertensive medication aiming at a BP goal <140/90 mmHg. For patients without documented CVD (CVD event or asymptomatic atherosclerosis) the SCORE calculator was used to distinguish between patients in need of primary prevention and those with no indication for CVD preventive measures. After

initiation of statins (atorvastatin, simvastatin, rosuvastatin, or pravastatin), the patients were followed until at least two lipid targets were
reached. Of the 426 patients referred to the Preventive Cardio-Rheuma
clinic, 63.4 % were in need of CVD preventive treatment, and secondary prevention was indicated in 77% of these patients. Achievement of
at least two lipid targets was successful in approximately 90% of all the
treated patients, using on average less than three consultations to obtain
these goals (Figure 5.1).

This high overall lipid goal attainment in patients with inflammatory joint diseases is encouraging, but whether it will sustain over time
is uncertain, considering the relatively low goal attainment of slightly
more than 40% reported in the general population [37]. Despite the presence of CVD, asymptomatic carotid atherosclerosis, or a calculated CVD
risk by SCORE ≥5%, a high proportion of inflammatory joint disease
patients did not receive recommended cardio-protective treatment at
referral date to the Preventive Cardio-Rheuma clinic. Ultrasound of the
carotid arteries revealed carotid plaques in approximately 50% of the

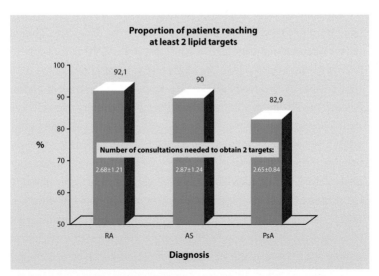

**Figure 5.1 Approximately 90% of the inflammatory joint disease patients in need of statin
treatment, obtained lipid goals in less than three consultations.** AS, ankylosing spondylitis; PsA,
psoriatic arthritis; RA, rheumatoid arthritis. Reproduced with permission from © BMJ Publishing
Group Ltd, 2013. All rights reserved. Rollefstad et al [36].

patients, which resulted in a correct stratification to indication for statin treatment with secondary CVD prevention lipid goals. Our results highlight the importance of performing carotid ultrasound during CVD risk evaluation in patients with inflammatory joint diseases.

In the general population there exists a linear relationship between lipid levels and risk of CVD [38]. Patients with inflammatory joint diseases have lower cholesterol levels compared with persons without inflammatory joint disease [35, 39, 40]. The complex interaction between inflammation and lipid levels has been investigated thoroughly [23,41–43]. Inflammation increases the risk of CVD in RA patients [44] but the corresponding low lipid levels may camouflage the actual risk for the executive physician. Patients treated with statins at the Preventive Cardio-Rheuma clinic, who obtained the guideline recommended LDL-c goal, were evaluated to reveal if baseline systemic inflammation (measured by CRP and ESR) and lipid levels were of importance regarding statin dose needed to obtain LDL-c targets [45]. Intensive statin dose was defined as rosuvastatin $\geq$20 mg and atorvastatin and simvastatin at the highest dose of 80 mg, and conventional lipid-lowering treatment was defined as all lower doses in accordance with the drug efficacy across doses obtained by the various statins in the STELLAR (the Statin Therapies for Elevated Lipid Levels compared across doses to Rosuvastatin) trial [46]. Change or up-titration of statins was done in cases of adverse events or failure to obtain LDL-c targets. Systemic inflammation or lipid levels at baseline were not associated with statin dose needed to achieve lipid targets (Figure 5.2).

Furthermore, there was no significant impact of anti-rheumatic medication (biologic and synthetic disease modifying anti-rheumatic drugs [DMARDs], prednisolone, and NSAIDs) on the relation between baseline lipid levels or systemic inflammation on doses of statins needed to achieve LDL-c targets. In a population-based cohort from US, patients with RA were less likely to obtain LDL-c goals in comparison with non-RA subjects, and that was related to an increased ESR at baseline [47]. Firstly, the relation between inflammatory parameters and lack of LDL-c goal attainment may reflect an increased RA disease activity resulting in lower compliance regarding both medications (statins) and primary care physician follow-up. Secondly, the low LDL-c goal attainment may reflect that this was a population-based cohort, where the patients were probably mostly attending primary care, and not results from a cardiology specialist practice as our Preventive Cardio-Rheuma clinic is. In the last case, patients attending such a specialist clinic might be more motivated and hence compliance will be better. In addition, a tight control regime was applied, which may not be possible in primary care. Thirdly, a limitation to the population-based report is that data regarding statin dose used in RA patients and non-RA persons are lacking. Interestingly, systemic inflammation at baseline was comparable for patients who did and did not obtain LDL-c targets in inflammatory joint disease patients attending the Preventive Cardio-Rheuma clinic. Thus, the mechanisms associated with individual statin response in the general population may also be applicable for patients with inflammatory joint diseases [48]. The data discussed suggests that systemic inflammation may be of limited value when developing individual lipid lowering CVD preventive strategies for patients with RA.

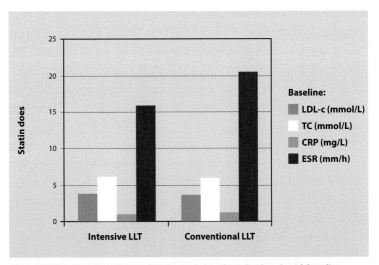

Figure 5.2 The association of dose of statin needed to obtain lipid goals with baseline lipids and systemic inflammation. CRP, C-reactive protein; ESR, erythrocyte sedimentation rate; LDL-c, low-density lipoprotein cholesterol; LLT, lipid-lowering treatment; TC, total cholesterol. Reproduced with permission from © BMJ Publishing Group Ltd, 2015. All rights reserved. Rollefstad et al [45].

Since effects of prospective randomized control trials with statins/ placebo on longitudinal CVD outcome are scarce, studies with surrogate CVD endpoints are of interest. In the ROsuvastatin in Rheumatoid Arthritis, Ankylosing Spondylitis and other inflammatory joint diseases (RORA-AS) study, we examined the development of carotid atheroma during 18 months of intensive statin treatment with rosuvastatin [49]. The aims were to evaluate change in carotid plaque height, and whether laboratory values or clinical parameters were predictors of the potential change in carotid plaques after 18 months of intensive lipid lowering therapy. The RORA-AS study was a prospective, open intervention study where 86 statin-naive patients with inflammatory joint diseases (RA: n=55, ankylosing spondylitis (AS): n=21, and psoriatic arthritis (PsA): n=10) who had carotid plaques were treated with rosuvastatin to obtain LDL-c goal ≤1.8 mmol/L. Carotid ultrasound was performed at baseline and after 18 months to evaluate carotid plaque height. Joint disease activity was assessed by the Disease Activity Score using 28 joints (DAS28) [50] and the Ankylosing Spondylitis Disease Activity Score (ASDAS) [51]. In order to address bone damage due to accumulated disease activity, digital X-rays of hands and feet were conducted and scored in accordance with the Sharp/van der Heijde method [52]. Compliance of rosuvastatin in the RORA-AS study was 97.9%. There was a significant reduction in both TC and LDL-c. The levels of the inflammatory biomarkers (CRP/ESR) and the composite disease activity values did not change during the study period. Intensive lipid lowering for 18 months induced carotid plaque height regression in patients with inflammatory joint disease (Figure 5.3).

The degree of atherosclerotic regression was inversely related to disease activity but was not influenced by LDL-c goal achievement, degree of change in LDL-c, or the LDL-c level exposure (area under the curve) during the study period. There was a significant difference in carotid plaque height reduction between patients using and not using biologic DMARDS (bDMARDs), in favor of non-users of bDMARDs. To date, there exist conflicting results regarding the impact of bDMARDs on the risk of future CVD. The analyses in the RORA-AS study were not adjusted for confounding by indication, which is a major concern because patients with the most severe rheumatic joint disease are more likely treated with bDMARDs, and they may also be more likely to have atherosclerotic disease as carotid plaques. However, demographic data, presence of CVD risk factors/co morbidities, disease activity, joint damage measured by the Sharp/van der Heijde method, laboratory values, and medication use

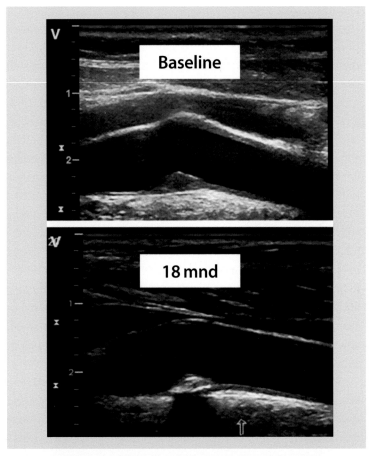

Figure 5.3 Carotid plaque at baseline and after 18 months rosuvastatin treatment.
Representative ultrasound images show an atherosclerotic plaque in the far wall of the bulb of the right carotid artery. At baseline, the plaque has a low density. After 18 months of rosuvastatin treatment, the height of the plaque is reduced and the density is increased, and calcification of the plaque has occurred (with acoustic shadowing below), reflecting stabilization of the plaque.
Reproduced with permission from © John Wiley and Sons, 2015. All Rights reserved.
Rollefstad et al [49].

at baseline were comparable for users versus non-users of bDMARDs. The increased risk of CVD in patients with RA has been related to joint disease activity, and our results indicate that disease activity may also influence the effect of anti-atherosclerotic treatment. Prospective randomized statin studies with clinical endpoints are warranted to reveal whether height reduction of asymptomatic carotid plaques will have an impact on future CVD events in patients with RA.

For practical purposes, statin initiation should be done as in the general population. A starting dose of statins that moderately lowers the lipids such as atorvastatin 40 mg daily is reasonable, and should be adjusted until lipid goals are achieved. Lipid targets for both primary and secondary prevention are presented in Table 5.3.

Anti-thrombotic treatment

As in the general population, the use of aspirin for the primary prevention of CVD events in patients with RA is not recommended, due to lack of reduction in CVD mortality as well as an increase in bleeding events [53].

The role of anti-rheumatic medications

Raised levels of high-sensitivity CRP have been found to predict CVD events in the general population [54]. Inflammation plays a key role in the atherosclerotic process and further in development of CVD. Large Phase III trials are being conducted in the general population with anti-inflammatory agents such as canakinumab (the CANTOS trial) and methotrexate (MTX; the CIRT trial) to reveal the effect on CVD endpoints [55]. Therapies aimed to reduce disease activity in RA may therefore also have a positive impact on the risk of CVD by reducing the

Treatment targets	Primary prevention	Secondary prevention
	NO CVD	CVD
	SCORE ≥5%	and/or SCORE ≥10%
Total cholesterol (mmol/L)	4.5	4.0
LDL-c (mmol/L)	2.5	1.8

Table 5.3 Treatment targets after statin initiation for both primary and secondary prevention of cardiovascular disease. CVD, cardiovascular disease; LDL-c, low density lipoprotein cholesterol; SCORE: Systematic COronary Risk Evaluation. Adapted from © Elsevier. All rights reserved. Perk et al [1].

systemic inflammation. On the other hand, adverse effects of diverse anti-rheumatic medication on CVD risk have also been observed.

Synthetic disease modifying anti-rheumatic drugs

The immunosuppressive drug MTX is standard medication as soon as the diagnosis of RA has been made [56]. Systematic literature reviews suggest that the use of MTX in patients with RA is associated with a decrease in the risk of CVD [57, 58]. The reduction in CVD related to MTX use may appear early in the joint disease course [59]. A window of opportunity may therefore also exist regarding prevention of atherosclerosis in addition to suppression of disease activity as a result of early initiation of MTX treatment. However, Greenberg et al did not reveal a cardio-protective effect of MTX in a large register study [60]. The impact of MTX on the lipid profile is still an unresolved question, as all studies addressing this subject [61–63] had a high risk of bias, according to a review performed by Westlake and colleagues [58]. Data on the effect of MTX on risk of CVD are all from observational studies, no randomized controlled trials have to date been performed, and it is not likely that such a study will be ethically justifiable to conduct considering the well-documented effect of MTX on the joint disease.

Biologic disease modifying anti-rheumatic drugs

The safety of tumour necrosis factor inhibitors (TNF-i), interleukin inhibitors, and other biologic agents has been investigated to some extent but controversies exist regarding the impact of bDMARDs on the risk of CVD in patients with RA. The adverse effects of TNF-i on lipid profile and fasting glucose levels are of particular concern [64, 65]. Systematic literature reviews have suggested that treatment with TNF-i is associated with a decreased risk of CVD [66, 67]. It has also been reported that TNF-i influence surrogate markers of CVD, such as aortic stiffness and carotid intima-media thickness [68]. The increase in lipid levels related to use of TNF-i may reflect a normalization of the lipids to the level the patient experienced prior to the RA disease [57]. Therefore, it is believed that these changes are likely to be due to the inflammatory-dampening effect of the drug. In a placebo-controlled study, atorvastatin was shown to significantly reduce tofacitinib-associated (a Janus kinase inhibitor) elevation of TC and LDL-c levels [69]. Responders to TNF-i seem to benefit the most with regard to risk reduction of CVD [70].

Non-steroidal anti-inflammatory drugs

In 2004, the cyclooxygenase-2 selective inhibitor rofecoxib was withdrawn from the market due to increased risk of CVD events associated with the drug [71]. Use of several NSAIDs has been reported to increase the risk of CVD in both observational and randomized trials [72-75]. However, naproxen seems to be the safest NSAID in terms of CVD risk [75]. It is currently advised that NSAIDs should be taken at the lowest effective dose for the shortest possible time considering both the CVD risk and the risk of gastrointestinal bleeding, but strict avoidance of NSAIDs among patients with RA, who also have presence of CVD risk factors, may not always be justified [76]. Indeed, Lindhardsen et al reported that the CVD risk associated with NSAID use in RA patients was significantly lower than in non-RA individuals [77].

Corticosteroids

There exist uncertainties regarding use of corticosteroids in patients with RA and the effect on CVD risk. Adverse effects of steroids have been thought to be related to elevation in lipids. However, some studies have also revealed beneficial effects of corticosteroids regarding cholesterol levels [78, 79]. Corticosteroids cause a mild increase in fasting glucose levels, but development of diabetes is rare in those with a normal glucose tolerance [80]. Studies from diverse diagnosis groups have reported adverse effects of corticosteroids on CVD outcome [81]. The adverse effects of corticosteroids seem to be dose dependent. Wei et al reported that high-dose corticosteroids (>7.5 mg daily) were associated with a threefold increased risk of CVD events [82]. For RA patients receiving a similar dose, the risk of CVD events was approximately five times increased. Davis and colleagues showed that in those exposed to glucocorticoids and being rheumatoid factor-positive, but not rheumatoid factor-negative, were at increased CVD risk [83]. A possible confounding factor may be that rheumatoid factor positivity is associated with more severe joint disease progression as well as extra-articular manifestations. Development of iatrogenic Cushing syndrome due to prolonged steroid treatment may be a marker of increased CVD risk [84]. In summary, whether the risk of CVD associated with use of corticosteroids increases or decreases remains unclear. A low dose of steroids to decrease disease activity in patients with inflammatory joint disease may be beneficial concerning the risk of CVD.

Hydroxychloroquine

The use of hydroxychloroquine has been reported from several studies to have both a favorable glucose- and lipid-lowering effect [85], but the influence on CVD morbidity and mortality remains unclear. Of note, hydroxychloroquine seems to have a cardio-toxic effect in some patients, and has been associated with an increased risk of cardiomyopathy [86].

References

1   Perk J, De BG, Gohlke H, et al. European Guidelines on cardiovascular disease prevention in clinical practice (version 2012): The Fifth Joint Task Force of the European Society of Cardiology and Other Societies on Cardiovascular Disease Prevention in Clinical Practice (constituted by representatives of nine societies and by invited experts). *Atherosclerosis.* 2012;223:1-68.
2   Peters MJ, Symmons DP, McCarey D, et al. EULAR evidence-based recommendations for cardiovascular risk management in patients with rheumatoid arthritis and other forms of inflammatory arthritis. *Ann Rheum Dis.* 2010;69:325-331.
3   Corrales A, Gonzalez-Juanatey C, Peiro ME, Blanco R, Llorca J, Gonzalez-Gay MA. Carotid ultrasound is useful for the cardiovascular risk stratification of patients with rheumatoid arthritis: results of a population-based study. *Ann Rheum Dis.* 2014;73:722-727.
4   Nurmohamed M, EULAR task force. EULAR Recommendations for Cardiovascular Risk Management in patients with Rheumatoid Arthritis and other Inflammatory Joint Diseases. Eular Recommendation Update on Cardiovascular Disease in RA. *Ann Rheum Dis.* 2015;74:9.
5   Han C, Robinson DW Jr, Hackett MV, Paramore LC, Fraeman KH, Bala MV. Cardiovascular disease and risk factors in patients with rheumatoid arthritis, psoriatic arthritis, and ankylosing spondylitis. *J Rheumatol.* 2006;33:2167-2172.
6   Whitworth JA. Adrenocorticotrophin and steroid-induced hypertension in humans. *Kidney Int.* 1992;37:S34-S37.
7   Snowden S, Nelson R. The effects of nonsteroidal anti-inflammatory drugs on blood pressure in hypertensive patients. *Cardiol Rev.* 2011;19:184-191.
8   Robert N, Wong GW, Wright JM. Effect of cyclosporine on blood pressure. *Cochrane Database Syst Rev.* 2010;CD007893.
9   Kellner H, Bornholdt K, Hein G. Leflunomide in the treatment of patients with early rheumatoid arthritis--results of a prospective non-interventional study. *Clin Rheumatol.* 2010; 29(8):913-920.
10 Roman MJ, Moeller E, Davis A, et al. Preclinical carotid atherosclerosis in patients with rheumatoid arthritis. *Ann Intern Med* .2006;144:249-256.

11 Cypiene A, Dadoniene J, Rugiene R, Ryliskyte L, Kovaite M, Petrulioniene Z et al. The influence of mean blood pressure on arterial stiffening and endothelial dysfunction in women with rheumatoid arthritis and systemic lupus erythematosus. *Medicina (Kaunas).* 2010;46:522-530.

12 Mancia G, Fagard R, Narkiewicz K, et al. 2013 ESH/ESC Guidelines for the management of arterial hypertension: the Task Force for the management of arterial hypertension of the European Society of Hypertension (ESH) and of the European Society of Cardiology (ESC). *J Hypertens* 2013;31:1281-1357.

13 Catapano AL, Chapman J, Wiklund O, Taskinen MR. The new joint EAS/ESC guidelines for the management of dyslipidaemias. *Atherosclerosis.* 2011; 217:1.

14 Baigent C, Blackwell L, Emberson J, et al. Efficacy and safety of more intensive lowering of LDL cholesterol: a meta-analysis of data from 170,000 participants in 26 randomised trials. *Lancet.* 2010; 376:1670-1681.

15 Brugts JJ, Yetgin T, Hoeks SE, et al. The benefits of statins in people without established cardiovascular disease but with cardiovascular risk factors: meta-analysis of randomised controlled trials. *BMJ.* 2009;338:b2376.

16 Mills EJ, Rachlis B, Wu P, Devereaux PJ, Arora P, Perri D. Primary prevention of cardiovascular mortality and events with statin treatments: a network meta-analysis involving more than 65,000 patients. *J Am Coll Cardiol.* 2008;52:1769-1781.

17 Ridker PM, Danielson E, Fonseca FA, et al. Rosuvastatin to prevent vascular events in men and women with elevated C-reactive protein. *N Engl J Med.* 2008;359:2195-2207.

18 Sattar N, Preiss D, Murray HM, et al. Statins and risk of incident diabetes: a collaborative meta-analysis of randomised statin trials. *Lancet.* 2010;375:735-742.

19 Ridker PM, Pradhan A, MacFadyen JG, Libby P, Glynn RJ. Cardiovascular benefits and diabetes risks of statin therapy in primary prevention: an analysis from the JUPITER trial. *Lancet.* 2012;380:565-571.

20 Jones PH, Davidson MH. Reporting rate of rhabdomyolysis with fenofibrate + statin versus gemfibrozil + any statin. *Am J Cardiol.* 2005;95:120-122.

21 Alsheikh-Ali AA, Trikalinos TA, Kent DM, Karas RH. Statins, low-density lipoprotein cholesterol, and risk of cancer. *J Am Coll Cardiol.* 2008;52:1141-1147.

22 Akkara Veetil BM, Myasoedova E, Matteson EL, Gabriel SE, Crowson CS. Use of lipid-lowering agents in rheumatoid arthritis: a population-based cohort study. *J Rheumatol.* 2013;40:1082-1088.

23 Toms TE, Symmons DP, Kitas GD. Dyslipidaemia in rheumatoid arthritis: the role of inflammation, drugs, lifestyle and genetic factors. *Curr Vasc Pharmacol.* 2010;8:301-326.

24 Soubrier M, Zerkak D, Dougados M. Indications for lowering LDL cholesterol in rheumatoid arthritis: an unrecognized problem. *J Rheumatol.* 2006;33:1766-1769.

25 Toms TE, Panoulas VF, Douglas KM, et al. Statin use in rheumatoid arthritis in relation to actual cardiovascular risk: evidence for substantial undertreatment of lipid-associated cardiovascular risk? *Ann Rheum Dis.* 2010;69:683-688.

26 Lindhardsen J, Ahlehoff O, Gislason GH, et al. Initiation and adherence to secondary prevention pharmacotherapy after myocardial infarction in patients with rheumatoid arthritis: a nationwide cohort study. *Ann Rheum Dis.* 2012;71:1496-1501.

27 De Vera MA, Choi H, Abrahamowicz M, Kopec J, Lacaille D. Impact of statin discontinuation on mortality in patients with rheumatoid arthritis: a population-based study. *Arthritis Care Res (Hoboken).* 2012;64:809-816.

28 McCarey DW, McInnes IB, Madhok R, et al. Trial of Atorvastatin in Rheumatoid Arthritis (TARA): double-blind, randomised placebo-controlled trial. *Lancet.* 2004; 363:2015-2021.

29 El-Barbary AM, Hussein MS, Rageh EM, Hamouda HE, Wagih AA, Ismail RG. Effect of atorvastatin on inflammation and modification of vascular risk factors in rheumatoid arthritis. *J Rheumatol.* 2011;38:229-235.

30 Ikdahl E, Hisdal J, Rollefstad S, et al. Rosuvastatin improves endothelial function in patients with inflammatory joint diseases, longitudinal associations with atherosclerosis and arteriosclerosis: results from the RORA-AS statin intervention study. *Arthritis Res Ther.* 2015;17:279.

31 Van Doornum S, McColl G, Wicks IP. Atorvastatin reduces arterial stiffness in patients with rheumatoid arthritis. *Ann Rheum Dis*. 2004;63:1571-1575.

32 Charles-Schoeman C, Khanna D, Furst DE, McMahon M, Reddy ST, Fogelman AM et al. Effects of high-dose atorvastatin on antiinflammatory properties of high density lipoprotein in patients with rheumatoid arthritis: a pilot study. *J Rheumatol*. 2007;34:1459-1464.

33 Bansback N, Ara R, Ward S, Anis A, Choi HK. Statin therapy in rheumatoid arthritis: a cost-effectiveness and value-of-information analysis. *Pharmacoeconomics*. 2009;27:25-37.

34 Kitas GD, Nightingale P, Armitage J, et al. Trial of atorvastatin for the primary prevention of cardiovascular events in patients with rheumatoid arthritis. *Arthritis Rheumatol*. 2015;67.

35 Semb AG, Kvien TK, DeMicco DA, et al. Effect of intensive lipid-lowering therapy on cardiovascular outcome in patients with and those without inflammatory joint disease. *Arthritis Rheum*. 2012;64:2836-2846.

36 Rollefstad S, Kvien TK, Holme I, Eirheim AS, Pedersen TR, Semb AG. Treatment to lipid targets in patients with inflammatory joint diseases in a preventive cardio-rheuma clinic. *Ann Rheum Dis*. 2013;72:1968-1974.

37 Kotseva K, Wood D, De BD, et al. EUROASPIRE IV: A European Society of Cardiology survey on the lifestyle, risk factor and therapeutic management of coronary patients from 24 European countries. *Eur J Prev Cardiol*. 2016;23:636-648.

38 Stamler J, Wentworth D, Neaton JD. Is relationship between serum cholesterol and risk of premature death from coronary heart disease continuous and graded? Findings in 356,222 primary screenees of the Multiple Risk Factor Intervention Trial (MRFIT). *JAMA*. 1986;256:2823-2828.

39 Peters MJ, Voskuyl AE, Sattar N, Dijkmans BA, Smulders YM, Nurmohamed MT. The interplay between inflammation, lipids and cardiovascular risk in rheumatoid arthritis: why ratios may be better. *Int J Clin Pract*. 2010;64:1440-1443.

40 Semb AG, Kvien TK, Aastveit AH, et al. Lipids, myocardial infarction and ischaemic stroke in patients with rheumatoid arthritis in the Apolipoprotein-related Mortality RISk (AMORIS) Study. *Ann Rheum Dis*. 2010;69:1996-2001.

41 Choy E, Sattar N. Interpreting lipid levels in the context of high-grade inflammatory states with a focus on rheumatoid arthritis: a challenge to conventional cardiovascular risk actions. *Ann Rheum Dis*. 2009;68:460-469.

42 Sattar N, McCarey DW, Capell H, McInnes IB. Explaining how "high-grade" systemic inflammation accelerates vascular risk in rheumatoid arthritis. *Circulation*. 2003;108:2957-2963.

43 Toms TE, Panoulas VF, Douglas KM, et al. Are lipid ratios less susceptible to change with systemic inflammation than individual lipid components in patients with rheumatoid arthritis? *Angiology*. 2011;62:167-175.

44 Myasoedova E, Crowson CS, Kremers HM, et al. Lipid paradox in rheumatoid arthritis: the impact of serum lipid measures and systemic inflammation on the risk of cardiovascular disease. *Ann Rheum Dis*. 2011;70:482-487.

45 Rollefstad S, Ikdahl E, Hisdal J, et al. Systemic inflammation in patients with inflammatory joint diseases does not influence statin dose needed to obtain LDL cholesterol goal in cardiovascular prevention. *Ann Rheum Dis*. 2015;74:1544-1550.

46 Jones PH, Davidson MH, Stein EA, Bays HE, McKenney JM, Miller E et al. Comparison of the efficacy and safety of rosuvastatin versus atorvastatin, simvastatin, and pravastatin across doses (STELLAR* Trial). *Am J Cardiol*. 2003;92:152-160.

47 Myasoedova E, Gabriel SE, Green AB, Matteson EL, Crowson CS. Impact of statin use on lipid levels in statin-naive patients with rheumatoid arthritis versus non-rheumatoid arthritis subjects: results from a population-based study. *Arthritis Care Res (Hoboken)*. 2013;65:1592-1599.

48 Thompson JF, Hyde CL, Wood LS, et al. Comprehensive whole-genome and candidate gene analysis for response to statin therapy in the Treating to New Targets (TNT) cohort. *Circ Cardiovasc Genet*. 2009;2:173-181.

49 Rollefstad S, Ikdahl E, Hisdal J, et al. Rosuvastatin-Induced Carotid Plaque Regression in Patients With Inflammatory Joint Diseases: The Rosuvastatin in Rheumatoid Arthritis,

Ankylosing Spondylitis and Other Inflammatory Joint Diseases Study. *Arthritis Rheumatol.* 2015;67:1718-1728.

50 Prevoo ML, van 't Hof MA, Kuper HH, van Leeuwen MA, van de Putte LB, van Riel PL. Modified disease activity scores that include twenty-eight-joint counts. Development and validation in a prospective longitudinal study of patients with rheumatoid arthritis. *Arthritis Rheum.* 1995;38:44-48.

51 Lukas C, Landewe R, Sieper J, et al. Development of an ASAS-endorsed disease activity score (ASDAS) in patients with ankylosing spondylitis. *Ann Rheum Dis.* 2009;68:18-24.

52 van der Heijde D. How to read radiographs according to the Sharp/van der Heijde method. *J Rheumatol.* 2000;27:261-263.

53 Seshasai SR, Wijesuriya S, Sivakumaran R, et al. Effect of aspirin on vascular and nonvascular outcomes: meta-analysis of randomized controlled trials. *Arch Intern Med.* 2012;172:209-216.

54 Ridker PM, Wilson PW, Grundy SM. Should C-reactive protein be added to metabolic syndrome and to assessment of global cardiovascular risk? *Circulation.* 2004;109:2818-2825.

55 Ridker PM, Luscher TF. Anti-inflammatory therapies for cardiovascular disease. *Eur Heart J.* 2014;35:1782-1791.

56 Smolen JS, Landewe R, Breedveld FC, et al. EULAR recommendations for the management of rheumatoid arthritis with synthetic and biological disease-modifying antirheumatic drugs: 2013 update. *Ann Rheum Dis.* 2014;73:492-509.

57 Choy E, Ganeshalingam K, Semb AG, Szekanecz Z, Nurmohamed M. Cardiovascular risk in rheumatoid arthritis: recent advances in the understanding of the pivotal role of inflammation, risk predictors and the impact of treatment. *Rheumatology (Oxford).* 2014;53:2143-2154.

58 Westlake SL, Colebatch AN, Baird J, et al. The effect of methotrexate on cardiovascular disease in patients with rheumatoid arthritis: a systematic literature review. *Rheumatology (Oxford).* 2010;49:295-307.

59 van Dongen H, van AJ, Lard LR, et al. Efficacy of methotrexate treatment in patients with probable rheumatoid arthritis: a double-blind, randomized, placebo-controlled trial. *Arthritis Rheum.* 2007;56:1424-1432.

60 Greenberg JD, Kremer JM, Curtis JR, et al. Tumour necrosis factor antagonist use and associated risk reduction of cardiovascular events among patients with rheumatoid arthritis. *Ann Rheum Dis.* 2011;70:576-582.

61 Park YB, Choi HK, Kim MY, et al. Effects of antirheumatic therapy on serum lipid levels in patients with rheumatoid arthritis: a prospective study. *Am J Med.* 2002;113:188-193.

62 Georgiadis AN, Papavasiliou EC, Lourida ES, et al. Atherogenic lipid profile is a feature characteristic of patients with early rheumatoid arthritis: effect of early treatment--a prospective, controlled study. *Arthritis Res Ther.* 2006;8:R82.

63 Dessein PH, Joffe BI, Stanwix AE. Effects of disease modifying agents and dietary intervention on insulin resistance and dyslipidemia in inflammatory arthritis: a pilot study. *Arthritis Res.* 2002;4:R12.

64 Gonzalez-Gay MA, Gonzalez-Juanatey C, Vazquez-Rodriguez TR, Miranda-Filloy JA, Llorca J. Insulin resistance in rheumatoid arthritis: the impact of the anti-TNF-alpha therapy. *Ann N Y Acad Sci.* 2010;1193:153-159.

65 Tam LS, Tomlinson B, Chu TT, Li TK, Li EK. Impact of TNF inhibition on insulin resistance and lipids levels in patients with rheumatoid arthritis. *Clin Rheumatol.* 2007;26:1495-1498.

66 Westlake SL, Colebatch AN, Baird J, et al. Tumour necrosis factor antagonists and the risk of cardiovascular disease in patients with rheumatoid arthritis: a systematic literature review. *Rheumatology (Oxford).* 2011;50:518-531.

67 Roubille C, Richer V, Starnino T, et al. The effects of tumour necrosis factor inhibitors, methotrexate, non-steroidal anti-inflammatory drugs and corticosteroids on cardiovascular events in rheumatoid arthritis, psoriasis and psoriatic arthritis: a systematic review and meta-analysis. *Ann Rheum Dis.* 2015;74:480-489.

68 Angel K, Provan SA, Fagerhol MK, Mowinckel P, Kvien TK, Atar D. Effect of 1-year anti-TNF-alpha therapy on aortic stiffness, carotid atherosclerosis, and calprotectin in inflammatory arthropathies: a controlled study. *Am J Hypertens*. 2012;25:644-650.

69 McInnes IB, Kim HY, Lee SH, et al. Open-label tofacitinib and double-blind atorvastatin in rheumatoid arthritis patients: a randomised study. *Ann Rheum Dis*. 2014;73:124-131.

70 Dixon WG, Watson KD, Lunt M, Hyrich KL, Silman AJ, Symmons DP. Reduction in the incidence of myocardial infarction in patients with rheumatoid arthritis who respond to anti-tumor necrosis factor alpha therapy: results from the British Society for Rheumatology Biologics Register. *Arthritis Rheum*. 2007;56:2905-2912.

71 Bresalier RS, Sandler RS, Quan H, et al. Cardiovascular events associated with rofecoxib in a colorectal adenoma chemoprevention trial. *N Engl J Med*. 2005;352:1092-1102.

72 Garcia Rodriguez LA, Tacconelli S, Patrignani P. Role of dose potency in the prediction of risk of myocardial infarction associated with nonsteroidal anti-inflammatory drugs in the general population. *J Am Coll Cardiol*. 2008;52:1628-1636.

73 Kearney PM, Baigent C, Godwin J, Halls H, Emberson JR, Patrono C. Do selective cyclo-oxygenase-2 inhibitors and traditional non-steroidal anti-inflammatory drugs increase the risk of atherothrombosis? Meta-analysis of randomised trials. *BMJ*. 2006;332:1302-1308.

74 McGettigan P, Henry D. Cardiovascular risk with non-steroidal anti-inflammatory drugs: systematic review of population-based controlled observational studies. *PLoS Med*. 2011;8:e1001098.

75 Trelle S, Reichenbach S, Wandel S, et al. Cardiovascular safety of non-steroidal anti-inflammatory drugs: network meta-analysis. *BMJ*. 2011;342:c7086.

76 Bhala N, Emberson J, Merhi A, et al. Vascular and upper gastrointestinal effects of non-steroidal anti-inflammatory drugs: meta-analyses of individual participant data from randomised trials. *Lancet*. 2013;382:769-779.

77 Lindhardsen J, Gislason GH, Jacobsen S, et al. Non-steroidal anti-inflammatory drugs and risk of cardiovascular disease in patients with rheumatoid arthritis: a nationwide cohort study. *Ann Rheum Dis*. 2013 [Epub ahead of print]; doi:10.1136/annrheumdis-2012-203137.

78 Svenson KL, Lithell H, Hallgren R, Vessby B. Serum lipoprotein in active rheumatoid arthritis and other chronic inflammatory arthritides. II. Effects of anti-inflammatory and disease-modifying drug treatment. *Arch Intern Med*. 1987;147:1917-1920.

79 Choi HK, Seeger JD. Glucocorticoid use and serum lipid levels in US adults: the Third National Health and Nutrition Examination Survey. *Arthritis Rheum*. 2005;53:528-535.

80 Olefsky JM, Kimmerling G. Effects of glucocorticoids on carbohydrate metabolism. *Am J Med Sci*. 1976;271:202-210.

81 Souverein PC, Berard A, Van Staa TP, et al. Use of oral glucocorticoids and risk of cardiovascular and cerebrovascular disease in a population based case-control study. *Heart*. 2004;90:859-865.

82 Wei L, MacDonald TM, Walker BR. Taking glucocorticoids by prescription is associated with subsequent cardiovascular disease. *Ann Intern Med*. 2004;141:764-770.

83 Davis JM, III, Maradit KH, Crowson CS, et al. Glucocorticoids and cardiovascular events in rheumatoid arthritis: a population-based cohort study. *Arthritis Rheum*. 2007;56:820-830.

84 Fardet L, Petersen I, Nazareth I. Risk of cardiovascular events in people prescribed glucocorticoids with iatrogenic Cushing's syndrome: cohort study. *BMJ*. 2012;345:e4928.

85 Hage MP, Al-Badri MR, Azar ST. A favorable effect of hydroxychloroquine on glucose and lipid metabolism beyond its anti-inflammatory role. *Ther Adv Endocrinol Metab*. 2014;5:77-85.

86 Joyce E, Fabre A, Mahon N. Hydroxychloroquine cardiotoxicity presenting as a rapidly evolving biventricular cardiomyopathy: key diagnostic features and literature review. *Eur Heart J Acute Cardiovasc Care*. 2013;2:77-83.

Chapter 6

Non-pharmacological interventions for cardiovascular complications in patients with rheumatoid arthritis

Eirik Ikdahl

Introduction

According to the World Health Organization (WHO), around three-quarters of all cardiovascular disease (CVD) events can be prevented by improving lifestyle-related CVD risk factors [1]. In patients with rheumatoid arthritis (RA), the relative impact of lifestyle-related risk factors on CVD outcome, including smoking, unfavorable body compositions, unhealthy diets, and physical inactivity, remain undetermined [2,3]. Nevertheless, most studies acknowledge that these four lifestyle-related risk factors entail significant negative consequences with regards to risk of CVD in this population [3].

Lifestyle-related CVD risk factors were essentially not included in the 2010 European League Against Rheumatism (EULAR) evidence-based recommendations for CVD risk management in patients with RA [4]. However, the authors recognized that lifestyle should be considered as a major CVD risk factor and argued that lifestyle changes should be recommended to all RA patients. It is expected that lifestyle interventions will be included in the updated EULAR recommendations, anticipated to be reported in 2016.

© Springer International Publishing Switzerland 2017
A.G. Semb (ed.), *Handbook of Cardiovascular Disease Management in Rheumatoid Arthritis*, DOI 10.1007/978-3-319-26782-1_6

RA patients' adherence to lifestyle interventions may be poor compared with pharmaceutical interventions, and achieving long-term lifestyle changes will often require a great deal of support from health personnel, friends, and family [5]. Support from health personnel can come in the form of motivational conversations with focus on detection and counteraction of barriers to successful implementation of lifestyle interventions. When necessary, one should also consider involving specialized health personnel, such as physiotherapists, nutritionists, or psychologists.

Smoking

WHO defines tobacco use as one of the largest public health threats the world has ever faced. Considering that one in three CVD events are attributable to tobacco use, smoking undoubtedly represents one of the most important preventable CVD risk factors [6]. Indeed, there is also convincing evidence that smoking cessation will effectively reduce the risk of CVD events back towards normal [7].

Smoking and cardiovascular risk in rheumatoid arthritis

Smoking is not only highly prevalent among RA patients; it actually represents a risk factor for development of RA disease [3,8]. Furthermore, RA patients who smoke have higher rheumatic disease activity and respond less well to common anti-rheumatic medications compared with non-smokers [9]. As in the general population, smoking in RA patients is associated with adverse effects on a wide range of surrogate CVD risk markers [10–13], and increased risk for future CVD [14–16]. In fact, a recent meta-analysis found that RA patients who smoke have 50% higher risk for CVD events compared with non-smokers [3].

Interventions for smoking cessation

Taking into account that the negative consequences of tobacco use in RA patients are twofold, smoking cessation appears to be an ideal intervention to kill two birds with one stone. Appropriately, rheumatologists appear to be keen on recording smoking status and delivering smoking cessation advice to these patients [17,18]. However, the international

QUEST-RA survey revealed that there is a huge potential for improvement concerning implementation of specific strategies/protocols for smoking cessation in rheumatology departments [18].

Counselling and other best-evidence methods to achieve smoking cessation are the only lifestyle interventions that are specifically mentioned in the 2010 EULAR recommendations for CVD risk management [4]. There is good evidence that even brief advice on smoking cessation is effective [19]. A 30-second algorithm to deliver smoking cessation advice to RA patients, based on the Ask, Advice, and Act (AAA) approach, has been developed by the UK National Health Service (NHS) [20]. An example dialogue illustrating this algorithm is presented in Figure 6.1.

More intensive smoking counselling has a superior effect compared with brief advice [19]. To increase the chances of success even further, one can also take advantage of the synergistic effects of combining counselling with nicotine (gum, inhalers, lozenge, nasal spray, and patches) and non-nicotine (Bupropion, Varenicline) medications [21].

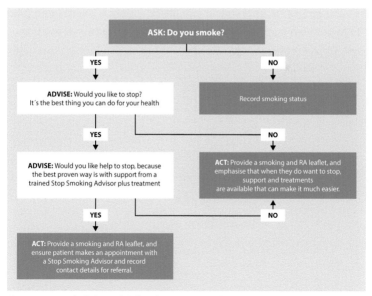

Figure 6.1 Example dialogue: brief smoking cessation advice to patients with rheumatoid arthritis. Reproduced with permission from © Helen Harris, National Health Service, 2014. All rights reserved. Harris et al [20].

When counselling to encourage RA patients to quit smoking, it is important to keep in mind that patients with chronic health conditions may face particular difficulties with regards to smoking cessation [22]. Identifying and neutralizing factors that are hindering this important lifestyle change are pivotal to reduce the risk of morbidity and mortality from CVD. It may be reasonable to base these discussions on the key barriers to smoking cessation in RA patients reported in a recent article by Aimer et al [23]:

1. Unawareness of association between RA and smoking
2. Smoking used as a distraction from pain
3. Unable to exercise as an alternative
4. Smoking used as comping mechanism for frustration of living with RA
5. Feeling unsupported and isolated from other RA patients

Weight control and body composition

From the general population, we know that individuals in higher weight ranges (ie, overweight and obese; Figure 6.3) are more prone to hypertension, hyperlipidemia and CVD events, as well as all-cause and CVD mortality [24].

- **Underweight: BMI is <18.5**
- **Normal weight: BMI is 18.5–24.9**
- **Overweight: BMI is 25–29.9**
- **Obese: BMI is ≥30**

$$BMI = \frac{Weight\ (kg)}{Height\ (m)^2}$$

Figure 6.2 Weight ranges by body mass index (BMI).

Weight and cardiovascular disease in rheumatoid arthritis

Approximately 60% of RA patients have a BMI over 25 (i.e. reaching the overweight or obese categories). This is comparable with that in the general population [25,26]. The prevalence of underweight in RA patients is most often reported to be around 2% [16,26].

The CVD risk imparted by being over and underweight in RA patients is a matter of debate. A recent meta-analysis revealed that obesity increases the risk of CVD morbidity in RA patients [3]. This is in line with several other studies that point to an association between high weight and hypertension, arterial stiffening, insulin resistance, and carotid atherosclerosis in RA patients [3,12,13,27]. However, numerous studies have reported that RA patients who experience weight loss and/or have a low BMI have the highest mortality risk [14,26,28,29], and in some of these studies obesity was protective against mortality [26,28].

It is believed that being underweight reflects higher levels of inflammation, which in terms of impact on CVD risk is more important than fat deposits [29]. It has also been argued that the explanation for these diverging results lies in the suggestion that the nutritional and metabolic state of patients with RA is poorly reflected by weight classes as defined by BMI. In this regard, the concept of rheumatoid cachexia (RC) has received great attention. RC is a state in which the relative amount of lean mass is reduced and the relative amount of body fat is increased. The prevalence of RC in RA patients may be as high as 20% and it is related to adverse effects on blood pressure, lipoprotein composition, and endothelial function [30–32]. BMI is not an optimal tool to detect RC, considering that the total body weight is not necessarily affected. To work around this, it has been proposed to reduce the BMI cut-offs for RA patients to 23 and 28 kg/m2 for those who are overweight and obese, respectively [33]. Waist circumference appears to be another viable option in clinical practice as it provides a good and easily measurable proxy for visceral fat deposits [30,34]. In the general population, waist circumference should not exceed 102 cm for men (ideal: 94 cm) and 88 cm for women (ideal 80 cm), although good evidence for these limits are lacking for RA patients.

Interventions for weight control in rheumatoid arthritis

Little is known about the CVD benefit that can be expected from weight control and improved body composition (ie, counteracting RC) in RA patients. However, there is no reason to believe that these changes will be less favorable than in the general population.

According to guidelines, there is strong evidence that lifestyle interventions to acheive weight loss in overweight/obese patients reduce the risk of Type 2 diabetes, improve lipid profile, and reduce blood pressure [24]. There is also evidence of moderate strength that weight loss in overweight/obese patients will reduce the need for cardioprotective drugs, and some evidence suggesting a reduction in mortality [24]. The remaining two subsections will deal with the two single most important non-surgical interventions to obtain weight control and improve body composition, namely healthy diets/nutrition and physical exercise [35].

Diet and nutrition

Dietary modifications have become mainstay of CVD prevention [35–38]. An issue related to dietary intervention studies is that they often attract big media attention than can make patients concerned [38]. When giving nutritional advice, it is important to emphasize that results from nutrition studies are often biased by inaccurate methodologies, confounders, and human memory [38].

Dietary interventions to reduce cardiovascular disease risk

The effect of dietary modifications in RA patients is generally vague, due to the fact that the available evidence largely stems from small, single studies with moderate-to-high risk of bias [39]. However, there exists some evidence that Mediterranean diets, fish oil supplements, and daily vegetable consumption may entail positive effects on various CVD risk markers in patients with RA [40–42].

Dietary guidelines/recommendations to reduce CVD risk often include basic concepts of a heart-healthy diet such as [24,35–37]:
- Food and nutrients to increase:
  - Fruits, vegetables, and whole grains
  - Low-fat dairy products

- Lean meat, poultry, and eggs
- Legumes
- Nuts and seeds
- Seafood
- Vegetable oils
- Foods and nutrients to reduce:
  - Solid fat: saturated and trans-fatty acids
  - Dietary cholesterol
  - Added sugars and refined grains
  - Sodium
  - Alcohol

There is sufficient evidence to conclude that variations of the heart-healthy diet (ie, the 'MEditerranean-style Dietary' [MED] approach and the 'Dietary Approaches to Stop Hypertension' [DASH] patterns) have beneficial effects on blood pressure and lipoprotein levels [35]. Furthermore, substituting saturated fats with unsaturated fats, carbo-hydrates, or protein will also entail significant benefits with regards to cardiovascular health [35].

Several 'quick fix' diets have become popular during recent decades, including high-fat, low-carbohydrate, high-protein, or intermittent fasting diets. However, the effect of these diets in terms of weight reduction appears to be largely short-term, and sustained weight control is still best achieved by securing an energy deficit [35,43]. An energy deficit is most commonly achieved by: (A) limiting energy intake per day (1200–1500 and 1500–1800 kCal/day for women and men, respectively); (B) estimating the energy requirements for the patient and prescribing an energy deficit (typically a deficit of 500–750 kCal/day, alternatively 30% energy deficit); or (C) ad libitum approaches, in which the energy deficit is rather obtained by restricting/eliminating particular foods [24]. It is important to discourage rapid weight loss with large energy deficits and complex/strict diets since they are harder to implement successfully and may put some patients at nutritional risk [39,43]. For some patients, it may also be advisable to involve a nutritional specialist.

Physical exercise

The inverse dose-response relationship between level of physical activity and risk of CVD is well established [35,44]. Eliminating physical inactivity would reduce the total number of coronary heart disease events by around 5%, and even more in populations with high CVD risk [45,46]. The mechanisms underlying the cardioprotective effects of exercise are not completely understood, although some researchers suggest that improvements in blood pressure and lipid profile (low-density lipoprotein cholesterol [LDL-c] in particular) account for around 50% [35]. Furthermore, there is also some evidence suggesting that the anti-inflammatory properties of exercise may play an important role [47].

Activity and inactivity in rheumatoid arthritis

Physical inactivity and low physical capacity are relatively common in RA [8]. Studies have indicated this is linked to RA disease-related barriers (ie, pain, fatigue, stiffness, and reduced mobility) in addition to fear-avoidance due to the perception that exercise may be harmful with regards to rheumatic disease activity and joint health [48]. In fact, the current consensus is that physical activity in RA patients may have both cardioprotective and anti-rheumatic properties [47,49]. More specifically, exercise may improve RA-related factors, such as health status, RC, pain, inflammation, fatigue, and overall joint health [47,49–51]; in addition to improving CVD risk factors, including endothelial function, blood pressure, lipoproteins, adiposity, and CVD risk calculator estimates [52,53]. However, more research is required to determine the effect of physical inactivity on hard CVD endpoints in RA patients [3].

Cardiovascular disease prevention by physical exercise

Although the EULAR recommendations for CVD risk management do not specifically recommend physical activity for RA patients, the authors do recognize that exercise is pivotal for CVD risk reduction in these patients [4].

There is a growing body of evidence regarding the safety and feasibility of endurance and resistance-type exercise for RA patients. For instance, walking represents a form of exercise that can be recommended for most RA patients, while patients with stable disease/medication can safely engage in moderate intensity exercise and resistance training [54–56]. In addition, progressive, high-intensity, low-impact aerobic and resistance exercise programmes appear to be feasible and do not cause adverse effects on large joint health [57,58].

The evidence-based exercise programme recommended by American College of Cardiology (ACC)/American Heart Association (AHA) to reduce CVD risk in the general population includes three to four sessions of moderate-to-vigorous intensity exercise per week, each session lasting on average 40 minutes [35]. An alternative exercise program recommended for RA patients was recently proposed in an article by Metsios et al (Table 6.1) [49].

There are some precautions that have to be considered before recommending physical exercise to RA patients. Firstly, there exists a hypothetical risk that high-impact weight-bearing exercises may injure joints, especially to those who have pre-existing damage. Although this risk has to date not been properly investigated, it is recommended that more strenuous exercise programs with high-impact stress are prescribed in collaboration with an experienced physiotherapist. Secondly, one should keep in mind that RA patients often have a low adherence to physicians' advice to engage in physical training and tend to overestimate their own level and frequency of physical activity [5,59]. To overcome these issues, it may be reasonable to determine possible barriers to exercise. It has been shown that many RA patients have 'arthritis-specific' barriers in addition to the traditional barriers to exercise (ie, age, high BMI, and lack of motivation) [48,60]. In a recent review, Veldhuijzen van Zanten et al found that pain and fatigue were the most common 'arthritis-specific' barriers while reduced mobility and stiffness were also common [48]. Interestingly, RA patients who engaged in physical activities regularly reported the same perceived barriers as those who were physically inactive, indicating that these barriers are not definitive [48].

One last precaution is related to the high frequency of subclinical atherosclerotic disease in RA patients as exercise may reveal symptoms of previously unrecognized conditions (eg, angina pectoris and peripheral artery disease). If this is the case, the symptoms must be evaluated by relevant health personnel before physical activity is resumed.

Month	Recommended exercise program
First month	
Evaluation of cardiorespiratory fitness, patient's preferences, and functional ability	• Frequency: three times/week, two out of the three of which are supervised (ie, cardiac rehabilitation center • Intensity: 60–75% of cardiorespiratory fitness. During the first month, the intensity can be kept at the lower end of the target heart rate • Type: Three circuits of three to four aerobic exercise in intervals of 3–4 minutes each using the following exercises: brisk treadmill uphill walking, stationary cycling, rowing on row-ergometer, and step climbing • Time: 10 minute warm-ups (five to six gentle stretching exercises), 30–45 minutes main session, and 10 minute cool down (gentle aerobic and stretching exercises)
Second and third months:	
In addition to the above, resistance exercises are incorporated in the exercise training at the end of every circuit	• Frequency: aerobic: same as above; resistance: once a week during the second month and thereafter twice a week. • Intensity: aerobic: same as above; resistance: 10–15 repetitions at 40–60% of one repetition maximum identified via a submaximal protocol (four to six repetitions) • Type: aerobic: same as above; resistance: five different exercises that correspond to five large muscle groups (leg press, chest press, shoulder press, back press, and abdominal exercises) • Time: 10 minutes warm-up (five to six gentle stretching exercises), approximately 60 minutes main session (with the addition of resistance training), 10 minutes cool down (gentle aerobic and stretching exercises)
After the third month	
	• Adjust/increase the intensity of both aerobic and resistance exercise based on the patient's performance and functional ability • Maintain adherence to the programme by providing support when needed, correct technique to avoid injury, and set up exercise-related targets to monitor

Table 6.1 Example of exercise program for patients with rheumatoid arthritis. Adapted from © Taylor & Francis Group, 2015. All rights reserved. Metsios et al [49].

References

1   World Health Organization. Global health risks: mortality and burden of disease attributable to selected major risks. WHO Library Cataloguing in Publication Data; 2009. http://www.who.int/healthinfo/global_burden_disease/GlobalHealthRisks_report_full.pdf. Accessed February 9, 2015.

2   Liao KP, Solomon DH. Traditional cardiovascular risk factors, inflammation and cardiovascular risk in rheumatoid arthritis. *Rheumatology*. 2013;52:45-52.

3   Baghdadi LR, Woodman RJ, Shanahan EM, Mangoni AA. The impact of traditional cardiovascular risk factors on cardiovascular outcomes in patients with rheumatoid arthritis: a systematic review and meta-analysis. *PLoS One*. 2015;10:e0117952.

4   Peters MJ, Symmons DP, McCarey D, et al. EULAR evidence-based recommendations for cardiovascular risk management in patients with rheumatoid arthritis and other forms of inflammatory arthritis. *Ann Rheum Dis*. 2010;69:325-331.

5   van Breukelen-van der Stoep DF, Zijlmans J, van Zeben D, et al. Adherence to cardiovascular prevention strategies in patients with rheumatoid arthritis. *Scand J Rheumatol*. 2015;44: 443-448.

6   Lightwood JM, Glantz SA. Short-term economic and health benefits of smoking cessation: myocardial infarction and stroke. *Circulation*. 1997;96:1089-1096.

7   Gellert C, Schottker B, Muller H, Holleczek B, Brenner H. Impact of smoking and quitting on cardiovascular outcomes and risk advancement periods among older adults. *Eur J Epidemiol*. 2013;28:649-658.

8   Brady SR, de Courten B, Reid CM, Cicuttini FM, de Courten MP, Liew D. The role of traditional cardiovascular risk factors among patients with rheumatoid arthritis. *J Rheumatol*. 2009;36: 34-40.

9   Serra-Bonett N, Rodriguez MA. The swollen joint, the thickened artery, and the smoking gun: tobacco exposure, citrullination and rheumatoid arthritis. *Rheumatol Int*. 2011;31:567-572.

10 Chung CP, Oeser A, Raggi P, et al. Increased coronary-artery atherosclerosis in rheumatoid arthritis: relationship to disease duration and cardiovascular risk factors. *Arthritis Rheum*. 2005;52:3045-3053.

11 Zampeli E, Protogerou A, Stamatelopoulos K, et al. Predictors of new atherosclerotic carotid plaque development in patients with rheumatoid arthritis: a longitudinal study. *Arthritis Res Ther*. 2012;14:R44.

12 Sliem H, Nasr G. Change of the aortic elasticity in rheumatoid arthritis: Relationship to associated cardiovascular risk factors. *J Cardiovasc Dis Res*. 2010;1:110-115.

13 Gerli R, Sherer Y, Vaudo G, et al. Early atherosclerosis in rheumatoid arthritis: effects of smoking on thickness of the carotid artery intima media. *Ann N Y Acad Sci*. 2005;1051:281-290.

14 England BR, Sayles H, Michaud K, et al. Cause-specific mortality in US veteran men with rheumatoid arthritis. *Arthritis Care Res (Hoboken)*. 2016;68:35-45.

15 Wolfe F, Michaud K. The risk of myocardial infarction and pharmacologic and nonpharmacologic myocardial infarction predictors in rheumatoid arthritis: a cohort and nested case-control analysis. *Arthritis Rheum*. 2008;58:2612-2621.

16 Zonana-Nacach A, Santana-Sahagun E, Jimenez-Balderas FJ, Camargo-Coronel A. Prevalence and factors associated with metabolic syndrome in patients with rheumatoid arthritis and systemic lupus erythematosus. *J Clin Rheumatol*. 2008;14:74-77.

17 Ikdahl E, Rollefstad S, Olsen IC, et al. EULAR task force recommendations on annual cardiovascular risk assessment for patients with rheumatoid arthritis: an audit of the success of implementation in a rheumatology outpatient clinic. *BioMed Res Int*. 2015;2015:515280.

18 Naranjo A, Khan NA, Cutolo M, et al. Smoking cessation advice by rheumatologists: results of an international survey. *Rheumatology*. 2014;53:1825-1829.

19 Stead LF, Bergson G, Lancaster T. Physician advice for smoking cessation. *Cochrane Database Syst Rev*. 2008:CD000165.

20 National Health Service. Smoking and rheumatoid arthritis: how to deliver brief smoking advice. http://www.nras.org.uk/data/files/For%20professionals/Smoking%20and%20RA/RA%20Smoking%20Brief%20advice%20leaflet1.pdf. Accessed February 9, 2015.

21 Phs Guideline Update Panel L, Staff. Treating tobacco use and dependence: 2008 update U.S. Public Health Service Clinical Practice Guideline executive summary. *Respir Care.* 2008;539:1217-1222.

22 Gritz ER, Vidrine DJ, Fingeret MC. Smoking cessation a critical component of medical management in chronic disease populations. *Am J Prev Med.* 2007;33:414-422.

23 Aimer P, Stamp L, Stebbings S, Valentino N, Cameron V, Treharne GJ. Identifying barriers to smoking cessation in rheumatoid arthritis. *Arthritis Care Res.* 2015;67:607-615.

24 Jensen MD, Ryan DH, Apovian CM, et al. 2013 AHA/ACC/TOS guideline for the management of overweight and obesity in adults: a report of the American College of Cardiology/American Heart Association Task Force on Practice Guidelines and The Obesity Society. *J Am Coll Cardiol.* 2014;63:2985-3023.

25 Naranjo A, Sokka T, Descalzo MA, et al. Cardiovascular disease in patients with rheumatoid arthritis: results from the QUEST-RA study. *Arthritis Res Ther.* 2008;10:R30.

26 Wolfe F, Michaud K. Effect of body mass index on mortality and clinical status in rheumatoid arthritis. *Arthritis Care Res.* 2012;64:1471-1479.

27 Stavropoulos-Kalinoglou A, Metsios GS, Panoulas VF, et al. Associations of obesity with modifiable risk factors for the development of cardiovascular disease in patients with rheumatoid arthritis. *Ann Rheum Dis.* 2009;68:242-245.

28 Escalante A, Haas RW, del Rincon I. Paradoxical effect of body mass index on survival in rheumatoid arthritis: role of comorbidity and systemic inflammation. *Arch Intern Med.* 2005;165:1624-1629.

29 Kremers HM, Nicola PJ, Crowson CS, Ballman KV, Gabriel SE. Prognostic importance of low body mass index in relation to cardiovascular mortality in rheumatoid arthritis. *Arthritis Rheum.* 2004;50:3450-3457.

30 Challal S, Minichiello E, Boissier MC, Semerano L. Cachexia and adiposity in rheumatoid arthritis. Relevance for disease management and clinical outcomes. *Joint Bone Spine.* 2015; doi:10.1016/j.jbspin.2015.04.010 [Epub ahead of print].

31 Elkan AC, Hakansson N, Frostegard J, Cederholm T, Hafstrom I. Rheumatoid cachexia is associated with dyslipidemia and low levels of atheroprotective natural antibodies against phosphorylcholine but not with dietary fat in patients with rheumatoid arthritis: a cross-sectional study. *Arthritis Res Ther.* 2009;11:R37.

32 Delgado-Frias E, Gonzalez-Gay MA, Muniz-Montes JR, et al. Relationship of abdominal adiposity and body composition with endothelial dysfunction in patients with rheumatoid arthritis. *Clin Exp Rheumatol.* 2015;33:516-523.

33 Stavropoulos-Kalinoglou A, Metsios GS, Koutedakis Y, et al. Redefining overweight and obesity in rheumatoid arthritis patients. *Ann Rheum Dis.* 2007;66:1316-1321.

34 Uutela T, Kautiainen H, Jarvenpaa S, Salomaa S, Hakala M, Hakkinen A. Waist circumference based abdominal obesity may be helpful as a marker for unmet needs in patients with RA. *Scand J Rheumatol.* 2014;43:279-285.

35 Eckel RH, Jakicic JM, Ard JD, et al. 2013 AHA/ACC guideline on lifestyle management to reduce cardiovascular risk: a report of the American College of Cardiology/American Heart Association Task Force on Practice Guidelines. *J Am Coll Cardiol.* 2014;63:2960-2984.

36 Perk J, De Backer G, Gohlke H, et al. European Guidelines on cardiovascular disease prevention in clinical practice (version 2012): The Fifth Joint Task Force of the European Society of Cardiology and Other Societies on Cardiovascular Disease Prevention in Clinical Practice (constituted by representatives of nine societies and by invited experts). *Atherosclerosis.* 2012;223:1-68.

37 Anderson TJ, Gregoire J, Hegele RA, et al. 2012 update of the Canadian Cardiovascular Society guidelines for the diagnosis and treatment of dyslipidemia for the prevention of cardiovascular disease in the adult. *Can J Cardiol.* 2013;29:151-167.

38 Sempos CT, Liu K, Ernst ND. Food and nutrient exposures: what to consider when evaluating epidemiologic evidence. *Am J Clin Nutr*. 1999;69:1330-1338.

39 Hagen KB, Byfuglien MG, Falzon L, Olsen SU, Smedslund G. Dietary interventions for rheumatoid arthritis. *Cochrane Database Syst Rev*. 2009:CD006400.

40 McKellar G, Morrison E, McEntegart A, et al. A pilot study of a Mediterranean-type diet intervention in female patients with rheumatoid arthritis living in areas of social deprivation in Glasgow. *Ann Rheum Dis*. 2007;66:1239-1243.

41 Olendzki BC, Leung K, Van Buskirk S, Reed G, Zurier RB. Treatment of rheumatoid arthritis with marine and botanical oils: influence on serum lipids. *Evid Based Complement Alternat Med*. 2011;2011:827286.

42 Crilly MA, McNeill G. Arterial dysfunction in patients with rheumatoid arthritis and the consumption of daily fruits and daily vegetables. *Eur J Clin Nutr*. 2012;66:345-352.

43 Malik VS, Hu FB. Popular weight-loss diets: from evidence to practice. *Nat Clin Pract Cardiovasc Med*. 2007;4:34-41.

44 Sattelmair J, Pertman J, Ding EL, Kohl HW 3rd, Haskell W, Lee IM. Dose response between physical activity and risk of coronary heart disease: a meta-analysis. *Circulation*. 2011;124:789-795.

45 Lee IM, Shiroma EJ, Lobelo F, et al. Effect of physical inactivity on major non-communicable diseases worldwide: an analysis of burden of disease and life expectancy. *Lancet*. 2012;380:219-229.

46 Taylor RS, Brown A, Ebrahim S, et al. Exercise-based rehabilitation for patients with coronary heart disease: systematic review and meta-analysis of randomized controlled trials. *Am J Med*. 2004;116:682-692.

47 Benatti FB, Pedersen BK. Exercise as an anti-inflammatory therapy for rheumatic diseases-myokine regulation. *Nat Rev Rheumatol*. 2015;11:86-97.

48 Veldhuijzen van Zanten JJ, Rouse PC, Hale ED, et al. Perceived barriers, facilitators and benefits for regular physical activity and exercise in patients with rheumatoid arthritis: a review of the literature. *Sports Med*. 2015. 2015;45:1401-1412.

49 Metsios GS, Stavropoulos-Kalinoglou A, Kitas GD. The role of exercise in the management of rheumatoid arthritis. *Expert Rev Clin Immunol*. 2015;11:1121-1130.

50 Jahanbin I, Hoseini Moghadam M, Nazarinia MA, Ghodsbin F, Bagheri Z, Ashraf AR. The effect of conditioning exercise on the health status and pain in patients with rheumatoid arthritis: a randomized controlled clinical trial. *Int J Community Based Nurs Midwifery*. 2014;2:169-176.

51 Hakkinen A, Pakarinen A, Hannonen P, et al. Effects of prolonged combined strength and endurance training on physical fitness, body composition and serum hormones in women with rheumatoid arthritis and in healthy controls. *Clin Exp Rheumatol*. 2005;23:505-512.

52 Stavropoulos-Kalinoglou A, Metsios GS, Veldhuijzen van Zanten JJ, Nightingale P, Kitas GD, Koutedakis Y. Individualised aerobic and resistance exercise training improves cardiorespiratory fitness and reduces cardiovascular risk in patients with rheumatoid arthritis. *Ann Rheum Dis*. 2013;72:1819-1825.

53 Metsios GS, Koutedakis Y, Veldhuijzen van Zanten JJ, et al. Cardiorespiratory fitness levels and their association with cardiovascular profile in patients with rheumatoid arthritis: a cross-sectional study. *Rheumatology*. 2015;54:2215-2220.

54 Baxter SV, Hale LA, Stebbings S, Gray AR, Smith CM, Treharne GJ. Walking is a feasible physical activity for people with rheumatoid arthritis: a feasibility randomized controlled trial. *Musculoskeletal Care*. 2015 [Epub ahead of print]; doi:10.1002/msc.1112.

55 Baillet A, Zeboulon N, Gossec L, et al. Efficacy of cardiorespiratory aerobic exercise in rheumatoid arthritis: meta-analysis of randomized controlled trials. *Arthritis Care Res*. 2010;62:984-992.

56 Baillet A, Vaillant M, Guinot M, Juvin R, Gaudin P. Efficacy of resistance exercises in rheumatoid arthritis: meta-analysis of randomized controlled trials. *Rheumatology*. 2012;51:519-527.

57 Law RJ, Saynor ZL, Gabbitas J, et al. The effects of aerobic and resistance exercise on markers of large joint health in stable rheumatoid arthritis patients: a pilot study. *Musculoskeletal care*. 2015;13:222-235.

58 Seneca T, Hauge EM, Maribo T. Comparable effect of partly supervised and self-administered exercise programme in early rheumatoid arthritis - a randomised, controlled trial. *Dan Med J.* 2015;62:A5127.

59 Yu CA, Rouse PC, Veldhuijzen Van Zanten JJ, et al. Subjective and objective levels of physical activity and their association with cardiorespiratory fitness in rheumatoid arthritis patients. *Arthritis Res Ther.* 2015;17:59.

60 van der Goes MC, Hoes JN, Cramer MJ, et al. Identifying factors hampering physical activity in longstanding rheumatoid arthritis: what is the role of glucocorticoid therapy? *Clin Exp Rheumatol.* 2014;32:155-161.

Chapter 7

Conclusions

Anne Grete Semb and Silvia Rollefstad

Cardiovascular disease (CVD) is the major cause of death in the general population, but there has been a large reduction in both mortality and morbidity of CVD since the 1970s. Although patients with rheumatoid arthritis (RA) have an increased risk of CVD, and a mortality gap between RA patients and the general population has been described, it is not known whether this will be so in the future.

Exploring therapeutic targets

Patients with RA are a high CVD risk patient group. This is unrecognized and models for increasing the awareness of this issue should be evolved. Furthermore, use of currently available risk calculators does not yield correct estimates for future risk of CVD in patients with RA. Therefore, there is an unmet need for development of an RA-specific risk calculator. Lastly, only scarce data regarding CVD prevention with lipid lowering treatment on hard CVD outcome exist, both regarding primary (TRACE-RA) and secondary prevention (post-hoc analyses from the combined IDEAL/TNT trials) in patients with RA. In relation to hypertension, it is not known whether anti-hypertensive treatment and blood pressure goals recommended for the general population are optimal for patients with RA. In addition, data suggest that there is an incremental improvement of CVD risk reduction by increasing reduction of blood pressure. This might also be so for patients with RA, but this needs to be evaluated.

© Springer International Publishing Switzerland 2017   107
A.G. Semb (ed.), *Handbook of Cardiovascular Disease Management in Rheumatoid Arthritis*, DOI 10.1007/978-3-319-26782-1_7

New medications to treat both indications

There are several new medications for CVD prevention, and the most promising at the moment is alirocumab/evolocumab (proprotein convertase subtilisin/kexin type 9 [PCSK9] inhibitors), which is recommended to patients with primary hypercholesterolemia who do not achieve lipid goals with statins. An interesting clinical indication is patients with statin intolerance, but until now alirocumab has only been tested in addition to statin medication.

The evolution of biological disease-modifying anti-rheumatic drugs (bDMARDs) has revolutionized outcomes for patients with RA, and almost abolished the crippling joint destructions so commonly previously seen in these patients. The newest generations of bDMARDs the Janus kinase (JAK) inhibitors seem promising but effects on CVD outcome are still unknown for both the conventional bDMARDs and the newer generation of these drugs.

Future outlook and overarching goals

During the past decades, anti-rheumatic treatment has been developing in addition to 'treat-to-target' and tight disease control strategies, which together have improved the outcome for patients with rheumatic disease immensely. Improved disease control may also be of importance for reduction of CVD in patients with RA. Therefore, future studies will reveal whether remission is the mission not only for joint disease but also for prevention of CVD in patients with rheumatoid arthritis.

The increased risk of CVD in RA patients has been known for decades and implementing this into clinical practice is one of the large challenges. The awareness of the high CVD risk in RA patients is low both among the patients themselves and among health personnel. In addition, CVD risk recording and risk evaluation is inadequate in RA patients. Furthermore, patients with RA are also undertreated with CVD preventive medication both in primary prevention and after they have had a CVD event. Therefore, the overarching goal for patients with RA should be that they will have a structured system for CVD prevention equal to that of other high-risk patient groups, such as those with diabetes mellitus, familial hypercholesterolemia, hypertension, heart failure, and chronic kidney disease. This includes specific risk algorithms, guidelines for CVD prevention, and specialized personnel; an example being diabetic nurses for patients with diabetes mellitus.

Printed in the United States
By Bookmasters